ISO 13485 for Engineers

Priscilla Browne

ISBN: 9798778002975

Imprint: Independently published

Forward

This book is written to provide Quality engineers, medical engineers, device engineers with a practical and insightful companion to understand ISO 13485, Quality Management system for medical devices. It provides a straight-to-the-point perspective which should assist in the interpretation of the standard and provide a benchmark for what is expected in the application of the standard and compliance for industry.

Table of Contents

PART 1 ISO 13485

Introduction to ISO 13485 — 5
  Directives and Standards — 7
  Competent Authorities — 8
  Notified Bodies — 8
  How ISO 13485 differs to ISO 9001 — 11
  ISO/TR 14969 — 11
  Terms /Definitions — 11
  Process Approach — 12
  Plan-Do-Check-Act (PDCA) — 13

Quality Management System — 14
  Introduction — 14
  Regulatory Requirements — 15
  Risk Based Approach — 15
  Changes within the QMS — 16
  Documentation — 18
  Quality Manual — 19
  Control of Records — 20

Management Responsibility — 20
  Management Commitment — 21
  Customer Focus — 21
  Quality Policy — 21
  Planning — 21
  Management Review — 22

Resource Management — 22
  Provision of resources — 22
  Human resources — 23
  Infrastructure — 24
  Work environment & contamination control — 24

Product realization — 26
  Planning of Product Realization — 26
  Design and Development — 28

Production and service provision 42
Ctrl of monitoring & measuring equipment 42

Measurement Analysis 43

PART 2 Good Documentation Practices
Introduction 44
Quality Management Systems 52

PART 3 Validation
Introduction 57
Equipment and Software Validation 60
Software Validation 62
Process Validation 74
Packaging Validation 82

Appendix 1
-Summary List of MDR 2017/745 Chapters, Articles and annexes

PART 1 ISO 13485

Introduction to ISO 13485

ISO 13485:2016 is an international standard for the quality management of medical devices. It is of value and applicable to a number of business areas that are involved in the various stages of a medical device and its product lifecycle. It may be applied by a design company, manufacturer, raw material supplier, calibration service, sterilization services or distributer. The scope of the standard covers:

- design and development
- production, storage and distribution
- installation
- servicing (if required)
- decommissioning and disposal

In particular, manufacturers of medical devices and typically mandated by regulatory bodies to comply with ISO 13484, and must demonstrate compliance and application of the standard subject to certification and an audit process.

FDA, 21 CFR Part 820 is another example of a Quality Management system. While its official designation is a Quality System (QS) it serves a similar purpose to ISO 13485- Quality management system for medical devices. However, there is an important distinction. 21 CFR Part 820 has a regulatory standing in the United states. While many competent authorities require the application of ISO 13485, the framework of ISO 13485 is a standard opposed to a regulation.

For a company to decide to adopt ISO 13485 as a standard, it requires commitment for senior management to support the process and to resource it not only at its inception into a company but also to maintain and sustain the quality management system into the future.A company or organisations size and organizational structures may determine if the standard can be implemented. However ultimately, if there is a regulatory requirement depending on the product, then it must be embraced in order to meet regulatory requirements.

Naturally, there are benefits from adopting a world renowned standard and certification opens many opportunities. At its core, IS0 13485 is a process that has improvement, monitoring, feedback and quality embedded into its clauses and requirements. These work to strengthen a company in terms of what it can achieve and also improving and maintaining a quality that meets the needs of customers and regulatory bodies.

The requirements within the International Standard are 'complementary' to the technical requirements for product in order to meet customer needs and intended uses and applicable regulatory requirements and deliver safety and performance.

Revised in 2016, ISO 13485:2016 "specifies requirements for a quality management system where an organisation needs to demonstrate its ability to provide medical devices and related services that consistently meet customer and applicable regulatory requirements."[1] The scope of the standard can apply to any organisation or company involved throughout the life-cycle of a product, including design and/or development, production, storage and distribution, installation, or servicing of a medical device and design and development or provision of technical or professional services. [1] International Standards Organisation, www.iso.org

The 2016 revision is designed to address recent developments in quality management and other updated regulations that relate to the industry. Improvements in the new version of the standard include broadening its applicability to include all organisations involved in the life cycle of the product, from the concept stage to end of life along with greater alignment with regulatory requirements and post-market surveillance including complaint handling.

ISO 13485:2016 is also used by suppliers or external vendors that provide QMS related management system services. Requirements of ISO 13485:2016 are applicable to organisations regardless of their size and regardless of their type except where explicitly stated. For any clause that is determined to be not applicable, the organisation records the justification as part of their certification and quality management system.

ISO 13485:2016 has 8 sections (or clauses) which include:

1 Scope
2 Normative References
3 Terms and Definitions
4 Quality Management System
5 Management Responsibility
6 Resource Management
7 Product Realisation

Directives & Standards

When it comes to regulated industries such as medical devices it is important to be familiar with some key terms and definitions and what they really mean. In this section, some key terms that are applied widely and relate to regulated industries include:

- Directives
- Standards
- Notified Body
- Competent Authority

Directives are legal requirements which must be met by manufacturers or other bodies within the industry. Directives are based on legislation and are issued at governmental level. It is important to note that standards such as ISO 13485 help companies meet the requirements set up in directives.

Standards are not always mandatory. However, they help manufacturers be compliant with directives/legislation. They also represent the current and best practice in the field of study/industry. Harmonised standards are European standards prepared under a mandate from the European Commission, referenced in the official journal, and drafted so that compliance with their requirements relates to one or more essential requirements of the directive. These standards have special status because, when a manufacturer can show that their products meet the requirements of the standard, there is a presumption that the product conforms to the essential requirements of the directive that is covered by the standard.

Competent Authorities

When it comes to medical devices, a competent authority is the legally delegated authority mandated to monitor compliance to directives and legal requirements within the industry. The competent authority has the power to grant and revoke licenses.

FDA (Food and Drug Administration) CFR Code of Federal Regulations – U.S.

JPAL (Japanese Regulations for Medical Devices) – Japan

HPRA (Health Products Regulatory Agency) - Ireland

MHRA (Medicines and Healthcare Regulatory Agency - UK

Notified Bodies

A notified body is a certification organisation which the national authority (the competent authority) of a member state designates to carry out one or more of the conformity assessment procedures described in the annexes of the medical devices directives. The Medicines and Healthcare Products Regulatory Agency is the UK competent authority under the three directives.

In Europe, EN ISO 13485:2016 (previously EN ISO 13485 2013) has facilitated companies meeting the requirements of: Directive 93/42/EEC on medical devices. This harmonised standard gives companies the "presumption of conformity" to complying with directives.

MDR 2017/745

The new European regulations on medical devices and in vitro medical devices were adopted on 05 April 2017 and came into force on 25th May 2017. Both these 2 new regulations replace and repeal Council Directives 90/385/EEC, 93/42/EEC Directive 98/79/EC and Commission Decision 2010/227/EU. Although adopted and in force, the new rules shall only apply after a 3-year transitional period, whereby regulations will enter into force in April 2020 for medical devices and for five years after entry into force (April 2022) for the Regulation on in-vitro diagnostic medical devices. The core goal of the new MDR rules and regulations is aimed at establishing a modern and robust EU legislative framework to ensure better patient safety and quality from manufacturers.

The revision of the legislation was necessary to consolidate the role of the EU as a global leader in the sector over the long-term and to take into account all technological and scientific developments in the sector. The new regulations will ensure:

> a consistently high level of health and safety protection for EU citizens using these products

> the free and fair trade of the products throughout the EU

> that EU legislation is adapted to the significant technological and scientific progress occurring in this sector over the last 20 years

Medical Device Coordination Group

The Medical Device Coordination Group (MDCG) is an expert group established by Regulation, (EU) 2017/745 on medical-devices and Regulation (EU) 2017/746 on in- vitro diagnostic medical devices. Members are experts representing competent authorities all EU countries. The MDCG provides advice and expertise, assisting the Commission/ EU in implementation of both regulations.

Article 103 (1) of Regulation (EU)2017/7451 establishes the Medical Device Coordination Group (MDCG). The MDCG is currently made up of 11 distinct working groups:

1. Notified Bodies Oversight, (NBO)
2. Standards
3. Clinical Investigation and Evaluation, (CIE)
4. Post-Market Surveillance and Vigilance (PMSV)
5. Market Surveillance
6. Borderline and Classification (B&C)
7. New Technologies
8. Eudamed – see the register of Expert Groups under the code E01309
9. Unique Device Identification, (UDI)
10. International Matters
11. In vitro diagnostic medical devices, (IVD)

In the United States, medical device manufacturers need to meet the requirements of 21 CFR Part 820 of FDA regulations, many companies will seek certification to the standard to support the exporting of products. In Australia, it is a regulatory requirement for manufacturers of medical devices to meet the requirements of ISO 13485. In Canada, certification to ISO 13485 is part of the regulatory requirements. The content of ISO 13485 is interpretive (not prescriptive) which gives a degree of scope in how the requirements are applied and met within a company. Note: ISO 9001 has requirements and themes relating to continual improvement and customer satisfaction. These have been modified for ISO 13485.

How ISO 13485 differs to ISO 9001

> Customer satisfaction (ISO 9001) is changed to Customer feedback for ISO 13485

> Extra requirements regarding procedures for ISO 13485

> Extra requirements for records ISO 13485 (e.g. retention)

> Continual improvement is restricted to continual improvement of the quality management system for ISO 13485

ISO/TR 14969

ISO/TR 14969 is a technical report that is used for guidance on the application and implantation of ISO 13485. It is recommended for those responsible for the role out of ISO 13485 within their organisation. The content of ISO/TR 14969 is based on several established organisations such as the GHTF, ISO and input from regulatory bodies.

Terms /Definitions

In the world of standards, there is particular terms and concepts that are important to understand. In fact, many standards will define terms, definitions, scope and concepts as a preamble to the technical detail and requirements.
> - "as appropriate"- it is deemed to be appropriate unless the organization can justify otherwise

- For requirements that are "documented", a process of establishing, implementation and and maintenance must be demonstrated

- the term "product" is used, it can also mean "service". Product applies to output that is intended for, or required by, a customer, or any intended output resulting from a product realization process.

- "regulatory requirements" is used when referring to any law applicable to the user of this International Standard (e.g. manufacturer)

- "shall" indicates a requirement

- "should" indicates a recommendation

- "may" indicates a permission

- "can" indicates a possibility or a capability

Process Approach

ISO 13485 is based on a process approach to quality management. A process is any activity that receives inputs and converts them to outputs. In turn, outputs from one process can be used as an input to the next process. For an organisation to function effectively, it has to identify and manage numerous linked processes (inter-related). One such example of separate processes but where linkage and interactions occurs is the product development process and risk management process. While companies may have separate procedures for both, during the lifecycle of a product, risk management features heavily. Furthermore, many processes impact other processes or downstream processes. The application of a system of processes within an organisation, together with the identification and interactions of these processes, and their management, can be referred to as the "process approach".

When used within a quality management system, such an approach emphasizes the importance of:

- understanding and meeting of requirements
- considering processes in terms of added value
- obtaining results of process performance and effectiveness
- improving processes based on objective measurement

Plan-Do-Check-Act (PDCA)

A methodology that instills a process approach is PDCA.

Plan
- plan the objectives and required processes to deliver results meeting customer requirements and organizational policies

Do
- implement the processes identified

Check
- monitor & measure processes and product against policies, objectives and requirements for the product

Act
- take actions to improve process performance

Quality Management System

Sections
General requirements (4.1)
Documentation requirements (4.2)
General (4.2.1)
Quality manual (4.2.2)
Medical device file (4.2.3)
Control of documents (4.2.4)
Control of records (4.2.5)

Introduction

Section 4.1 of ISO 13485 sets out some general requirements of the quality management system. The requirement of the quality management system as something that is an ongoing process and system that is maintained is fundamental. If an organization decides to pursue compliance to the standard, they should understand it is not a one-time activity or project that has an end date or final output. Therefore, the wording in the general requirements states that the quality management system must be:

- ➢ Established
- ➢ Implemented
- ➢ Maintained
- ➢ Demonstrate its effectiveness

The organisation must implement a Quality Management System, or QMS in order to provide the framework and structure to achieve ISO 13485 roll-out and implementation. However, the role of the QMS does not stop there. After initial roll-out, the requirements of the standard must be maintained and determined to be effective on an on-going basis. The following processes should be documented:

- List of all processes
- Process interactions
- Monitoring of processes
- Resources to facilitate rollout of processes
- Measure and monitor effectiveness
- System of identifying improvements

Regulatory Requirements

Within the General requirements section (4.1), the term 'applicable regulatory requirements' is used 5 times alongside the requirements of the international standard (ISO 13485). This is a powerful and important element of the general requirements. "Applicable regulatory requirements' is a broad statement and in that respect places a degree of responsibility on the organization adopting the standard. It is indicating that the organization must also apply related regulatory requirements (e.g. legal, FDA requirements, EU MDR requirements etc).

Risk Based Approach

Risk management involves the systematic application of management policies, practices and procedures that identify, analyse, control and monitor risk. For a Risk Based approach to be applied to changes or a QMS system, a number of tools are required. Firstly, what is meant by a risk-based approach? It means that when any changes are proposed, they are assessed for the impact on the process and product and any risks are identified and mitigated.

The process of completing a risk assessment for changes to product or indeed the QMS, ensure that potential risks and risk scenarios are identified and evaluated. When the risks are known, mitigations and actions can be taken to eliminate the risks or to control them. The last line of defense should be detection (after elimination or risks)

For successful risk-based approach within a QMS, a procedure or SOP on risk management is typically available within manufacturing companies. This should clearly describe the risk management process and the various risk assessment tools, their application and guidance on how to complete them. The content of any risk management procedure or SOP should align with ISO 14971:2007 Medical Devices - Application of Risk Management to Medical Devices. Controlled templates for PFMEAs etc. also bring consistency and continuity to the process.

Changes within the Quality Management System

The quality management system shall be subject to change over time. Changes may be a result of continuous improvement, change in products, change to technology used and regulatory changes to name some. The standard requires changes in the QMS to be managed by the organization of company with the following considerations:

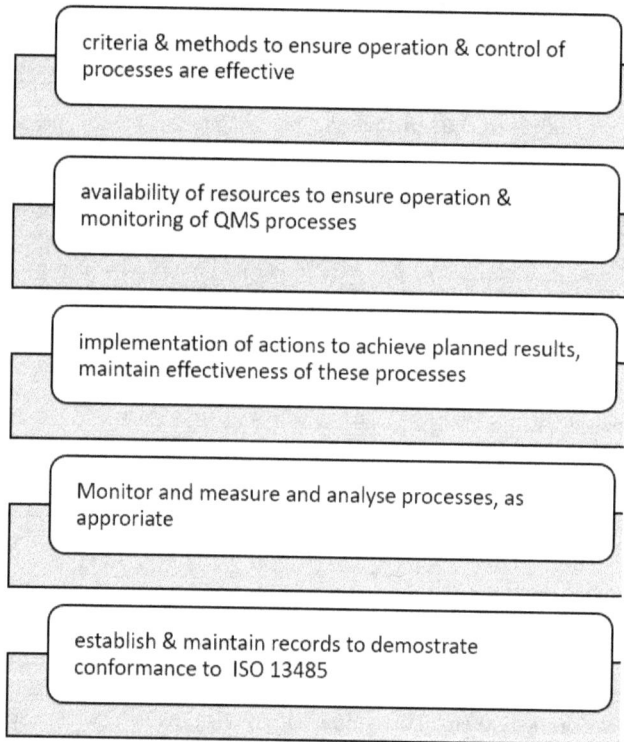

In addition, changes to the QMS must meet any applicable regulatory requirements. So, any legislation of regulatory requirements that a particular region or competent authority may require. (FDA 21 CFR 820, MDR 745/2015

Finally, in respect to changes to processes, they must be evaluated for any impact on the quality management process and also any impact on the medical devices / products produced within the quality management system.

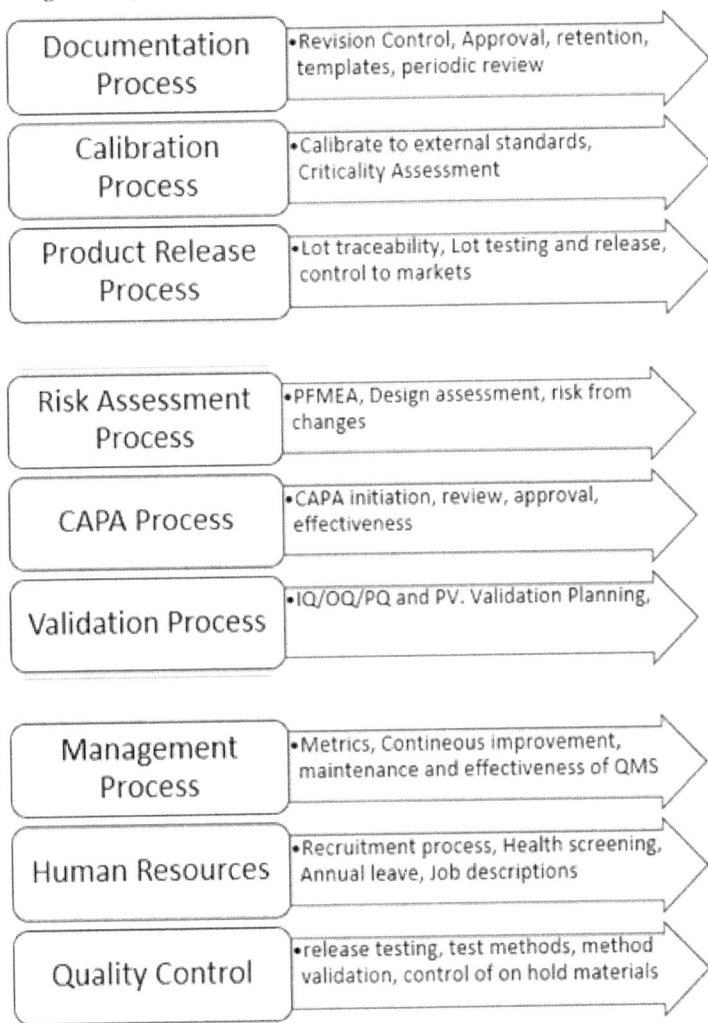

| Laboratory Process | • Purified water, raw materials testing, finished product testing |
| Incoming Materials | • CofAs, training, acceptance specifications, on hold, traceability |

Documentation

When it comes to the regulated industries such as the medical device industry, every process and procedure must be documented. Documentation ensures that everyone is working in the same manner with the same procedures. However, documentation is more than just writing down procedures and processes. It is also concerned with how documents are controlled, how they are updated and how they are stored.

Electronic Document Management Systems:

Electronic document management systems aka EDMS are now the norm and gold standard for most medium to large organisations. Many companies that provide medical device manufacturers with an EDMS can customise the system to match the business processes particular to an organisation. With configurable or customisable software, validation and proper verification is important to ensure the system operates as intended. There are also regulatory requirements that stipulate the expectations and requirements of such systems. For example, the application of electronic signatures and the presence of audit trials. FDA 21 CRF Part 11 details the requirements with regards to electronic records and electronic signatures. For medicinal products in Europe, GMP V4 Annex 11 specifies similar requirements.

Changes and Updates to Documents:

Revision control is a key element of the Quality Management Systems in place in regulated industries. As the need for changes in the document arises, the controlled document can be amended/updated. With each update the version number revises also. Some companies will use alphabetic revision control and to a lesser extent numeric revision control (Version A, Version B or Version 01, Version 02). Controlled documents should always have a version number or revision number electronically on each page of the document. This is similar to books which always list what edition they are. e.g. first edition or second edition.

Records:

Records are generated through the application of processes and procedures. These records can be related in quality inspection and manufacturing. The integrity and quality of records relating to the manufacture of medical devices is important, as it plays a part in safeguarding the patient or user. Records may also help in the investigation of any quality issues, complaints or adverse events that may arise. or GDP should be applied to records. In particular, handwritten entries should always be accompanied by a signature and date. This is important as traceability must be maintained in the event of an issue or complaint.

Quality Manual

The requirement for a quality manual requires (1) scope of QMS, documented procedures for the QMS (3) describe how the QMS and other processes work together. The structure of documentation is normally addressed in the Quality Manual. For example, Directives may be the principle quality document followed by standard operating procedures and then followed by work instructions.

Document Retention

Document retention time should take into consideration:

1) period of time the medical device is expected to be in the marketplace
2) legal considerations including liability
3) need or advisability of keeping documents indefinitely
4) retention time of related records
5) spare parts availability

Retirement of Obsoletion

- ➤ Good practice to retain one copy of obsolete controlled documents

- A minimum retention period should be applied. Regulatory requirements for longer retention periods should be understood.
- The company must apply suitable identification to obsolete documents

Control of records

Records are necessary to demonstrate the ongoing effectiveness of the QMS and as a means of providing evidence. Procedures must be in place to document how records and issued, approved, reviewed, stored, retrieved, identified and reviewed.

Records must also remain legible readily identifiable and retrievable. This requires electronic records to be maintained securely over time. Obsoletion of software that reads records can be of concern. For hard copy records, suitable achieving should be maintained. Furthermore, records must be available for review and have a retention period defined.

Management Responsibility

Sections
5.1 Management commitment
5.2 Customer focus
5.3 Quality policy
5.4 Planning
5.5 Responsibility, authority and communication
5.6 Management review

Management Commitment

It is essential that top management have an authentic and tangible commitment to meeting regulations and the expectations of customers. Quality should be at the forefront of all of activities. Management should encourage discourse and communication on all matters relating to internal processes, quality and the QMS as a whole.

Customer Focus

Customer feedback is a requirement of ISO 13485 and as such the manufacturer must engage with the customer. In instances where a defective product is received, the manufacturer must have a complaints process to facilitate proper feedback, communication and investigation.

Quality Policy

A Quality Policy has several purposes that an organization must cover. The policy sets out the organizations commitment to quality. Commitment is a fundamental principle which is intended to ensure quality is a ongoing theme for the company and not just a once off activity.

The policy should touch upon customer requirements, regulatory requirements and set out the core objectives and goals of the company. Commitment must be demonstrated from top management. Often a signed and approved quality policy is displayed by companies in its reception of hosting area.

Planning

ISO 13485 requires quality objectives for the quality management system but also for medical devices and any services that may apply.

Typical inputs into quality management system planning include
- quality policy
- quality objectives
- regulatory requirements
- quality management system standards
- Quality metrics (CAPA, NC)
- Business Metrics

Management review

The purpose of management review is to ensure the effectiveness of the QMS. Inputs to management review include:
(a) Audit results
(b) Customer feedback

(c) Process performance and conformity
(d) Corrective and preventative actions
(e) Deviations
(f) Regulatory changes and revisions

Management review should be ongoing and subject to reporting against the goals and objectives of the company.

Resource Management

Sections
Provision of resources (6.1)
Human resources (6.2)
Infrastructure (6.3)
Work environment and contamination control (6.4)

Provision of Resources

Resources is a broad term but refers to the
- People
- Infrastructure
- Suppliers
- Financial resources

A lifecycle approach is needed to maintain resources, so they are effective and suitable over the long term. Infrastructure must be properly serviced and maintained. People power is subject to retention and people moving industry and retirement. These scenarios all place pressure on resources and therefore must be given appropriate attention.

Human resources

Skilled and suitability qualified people play a key part in the maintenance and effectiveness of a Quality Management System. Some examples of personnel whose work requires them to be present in the work environment include:

- manufacturing team members and managers

- engineers
- material handlers
- quality engineers
- service suppliers or contractors
- maintenance personnel

Training Checklist:

- Suitable level in line with responsibilities
- Training is Documented and recorded
- Effectiveness of training
- Methods used to determine effectiveness
- Content of training kept current

Infrastructure

Equipment
- Equipment must meet the intended use and be designed, constructed, correctly installed and located to facilitate proper operation, maintenance and cleaning

Production
- Specifications that detail any allowable tolerances of production, measurement and testing should be documented and available for production personnel

Documentation
- Documented procedures should be available for the maintenance, cleaning and checking of all equipment used in production, and for the control of the work environment

Maintenance
- The determination of the necessary adjustments and maintenance intervals should be established.

Facility
- The organization should ensure that the buildings utilized are of suitable design and contain adequate space to facilitate cleaning, maintenance and other necessary operations.

Work Environment and Contamination Control

The work environment is closely related to infrastructure within a given organisation and they can both affect or impact upon the quality of products manufactured. Risk to product quality and patients is minimised by understanding the work environment and how it can impact the product. When the interactions and risks are understood, work can then be done to eliminate risks or at least control or monitor them. Environmental conditions that can impact upon product quality include:

- Humidity/ Relative Humidity
- Air Temperature
- Air quality

> Room pressure differentials (negative / positive)
> Air flow/velocity

The purpose of setting out requirements for the work environment is to ensure product is manufactured in a suitable environment that will assure the performance and safety of the medical device- *a device that meets the quality specifications*. Product quality can be influenced by the work environment, with the 3 most impactful been:

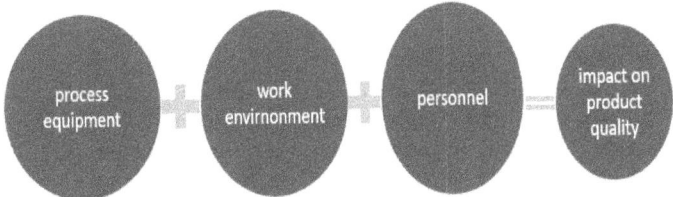

Product realization

Sections
Planning of product realization 7.1
Customer-related processes 7.2
Design and development 7.3
Purchasing 7.4
Production and service provision 7.5
Control of monitoring and measuring equipment 7.6

Product realization per ISO 13485 is the process of planning product development and introduction but also the subsequent steps that are meaningful in the success of the product introduction. Planning should be initiated early-on in the design stage and should include timelines, resources required, intended markets. One of the most important aspects of planning is gaining the correct stakeholder needs. Again these can be made up of various different inputs. Intended use of the device, will the device be disposable, who is the likely users of the device and so on.

Product realization must establish customer requirements and document the design and development efforts. ISO 13485 also has requirements around purchasing, production, service product and monitoring and measuring equipment.

- *Planning*
- *Customer Requirements*
- *Design & Development*
- *Purchasing Controls*
- *Production and service provision*
- *Control of monitoring and measuring equipment*

Planning of Product Realisation

Product realisation can be defined as a collection of processes and body of work that delivers a product or service to the customer. Remember, when it comes to medical devices, customers can be patients or users such as doctors and nurses. It should be noted that organisations can opt to exclude specific requirements, in cases where product realisation is not applicable. However, any such exclusion should be based on sound rationale with the case clearly documented. An example of this may be where design and development is not conducted by the manufacturer e.g. contract manufacturers.

Planning is an often underestimated but remains a key element of product realisation. If adequate time and resources are given to planning, it makes all other processes run smoother, and therefore should help to produce improved products and services.

With regard to customer communication, it is important to remind ourselves that we are concerned with ISO 13485 which as we very well know by now is the standard for medical devices. Therefore, having the right information available to the customer, patient or end user is important. When additional information needs to be transmitted or updates to information need to be communicated, an advisory note can be issued. Another important aspect of customer communication is customer feedback. This communication can be made up of positive feedback from the customer or users, or when there is a query with regard to a product or service. Therefore, processes or systems must be in place to make communication between customer and company both effective and timely.

Design and Development

Design and Development Verification and Validation ensure that the product is designed, developed and subsequently manufactured meeting all the customer requirements, regulatory requirements and business requirements. These requirements are classed as inputs to the design and development, and verification and validation ensure the inputs have been adequately taken into account. The design and development testing sometimes replicate the commercial applications of the medical device, hence providing a realistic challenge in order to have confidence in the medical device. Design controls are an important component of the FDAs Quality System Regulation, 21 CFR Part 820. Design controls apply to a wide variety of devices with varying levels of complexity. the regulation does not prescribe the practices that must be used, rather it establishes a framework that manufacturers must use when developing and implementing design controls. Such requirements much be appropriate to ensure that regulation allows design controls to be flexible enough to meet individual manufacturers own design and development processes.

Design controls are a collection of practices and procedures that are incorporated into the design and development process for a product such as a medical device. Based upon quality assurance and engineering principles, they provides a structure and clear path from user needs assessment to product delivery through a step-by-step process. Design controls ensure proper assessment of the design is completed during the design and development phase. It highlights technical issues, conflicts or deficiencies in design input requirements and allows them to be addressed early on in the process. Fixing a design issue early on reduces the cost of doing so at a later point and ensures the resultant design is appropriate for its intended use. Bringing a formal review process (design control) to the table assists engineers and managers in engaging with decisions and understanding them better. It also ensures that when future changes are made, they are documented and reviewed adequately with proper consideration to the design inputs. Design controls are a requirement of quality systems such as 21 CFR Part 820 (medical devices), and for certain classes of devices and per ISO 13485 - Quality Management Systems.

Benefits of Design Control:
- The intended use of the device is documented and approved
- It ensures inputs align with outputs
- Problems with designs or manufacturability are recognised earlier
- It creates a design "standard" and a "process" to allow benchmarking and consistency within an organisation

The development process depicted in the example is a traditional waterfall model. The design proceeds in a logical sequence of phases or stages. Basically, requirements are developed, and a device is designed to meet those requirements. The design is then evaluated, transferred to production, and the device is manufactured. In practice, feedback paths would be required between each phase of the process and previous phases, representing the iterative nature of product development. However, this detail has been omitted from the figure to make the influence of the design controls on the design process more distinct. The importance of the design input and verification of design outputs is illustrated by this example. When the design input has been reviewed and the design input requirements are determined to be acceptable, an iterative process of translating those requirements into a device design begins. The first step is conversion of the requirements into system or high-level specifications. Thus, these specifications are a design output. Upon verification that the high-level specifications conform to the design input requirements, they become the design input for the next step in the design process, and so on.

This basic technique is used repeatedly throughout the design process. Each design input is converted into a new design output; each output is verified as conforming to its input; and it then becomes the design input for another step in the design process. In this manner, the design input requirements are translated into a device design conforming to those requirements.

Clause 7.3 of ISO 13485 specifies the requirements for design and development of devices as part of the product realisation process. It should be noted that organisations can opt to exclude specific requirements of ISO 13485, in cases where product realisation is not applicable. However, any such exclusion should be based on sound rationale with the technical case clearly documented. An example of this may be where design and development are not conducted by the manufacturer e.g. contract manufacturers. Clause 7 (product realisation) of ISO 13485 details requirements for design and development controls. Clause 7 includes the following subparts:

ISO 13485 (Design and development) comprises:

Design and Development Planning 7.3.1
Design and Development Inputs 7.3.2
Design and Development Outputs 7.3.3
Design and Development Review 7.3.4
Design and Development Verification 7.3.5
Design and Development Validation 7.3.6
Control of Design and Development Changes 7.3.7

Design controls can be applied to any product development process. When the design input has been reviewed and the design input requirements are determined to be acceptable, the process of creating the device design begins. Product specifications are drafted and compared to the design input requirements. They then become the input for the next step in the design process. In the development and drafting of product specifications (e.g. critical quality attributes etc.) due regard must be given to product standards and industry best practices such as ISO and ASTM bodies. For example a catheter manufacturer should develop products with reference to ISO 10555 - intravascular catheters - sterile and single.

The term "phase approach" is often used when describing the design control process. It simply means that a sequence of tasks needs to be completed, reviewed and approved during the development cycle of a product or medical device. Tasks are grouped into phases or stages. At the beginning, technical issues relating to design input requirements may need to be addressed with solutions identified. Often a range of solutions can be available, utilising different technologies. These different solutions then go on to be reviewed at the design selection process. At design selection, the project team must choose and justify a particular solution. The next phase (such as design verification and validation) ensures that the design is transferred to product launch and commercial supply - no oversights or deviations in the design intent occur. It also ensures that the device meets the user needs and intended uses (design inputs).

A phase review is a process of evaluating the progress against the goals and activities of a particular phase. The phase review is typically completed at the end of each phase, but there may be a need to complete interim reviews for long or complex projects. For example, a design phase review is completed to ensure that the design input requirements make sense before they are interpreted into design specifications (design inputs phase review).

Changes made during design control are managed via document control procedures. For products built for commercial sale, the change management process is used to document and manage changes to the validated state of the process or the design of the product itself. While there may be more "flexibility" to make changes during the design phase of a project, diligence must be applied to any proposed change. Changes should be assessed by a multidisciplinary team with a management review.

An example of this is an exposure control system for a general-purpose x-ray system. The control function was allocated to software. Late in the development process, risk analysis of the system uncovered several failure modes that could result in overexposure to the patient. Because the problem was not identified until the design was near completion, an expensive, independent, back-up timer had to be added to monitor exposure times.

In addition to procedures and work instructions necessary for the implementation of design controls, policies and procedures may also be needed for other determinants of device quality that should be considered during the design process. The need for policies and procedures for these factors is dependent upon the types of devices manufactured by a company and the risks associated with their use. Management with executive responsibility has the responsibility for determining what is needed.

Design and Development Planning

It is the manufacturer's responsibility to establish and maintain plans that describe or reference the design and development activities and define responsibilities for implementation. The plans should identify and describe the interaction with different groups or activities that are part of the design and development process. The maintenance of plans to reflect an accurate state as the design and development progresses is also a key factor. The design and development planning is intended to be prospective in nature. It allows risks to be identified earlier and promotes timely delivery of projects.

The following is a list of key considerations to include in the design and development plan:

- Product Description, Goals & Objectives
- Markets intended for Launch
- Procedures & Records required by D&D process and Quality Management system
- Identify key tasks and activities
- Schedule and timing of tasks
- Details on verifications, validation and production requirements
- Risk Management Activities

Design Inputs

The aim of the Design Input stage is to (1) define, identify and document the user needs, the intended use and other design criteria, materials and process requirements of the medical device. These are broadly known as stakeholder needs and (2) translate these stakeholder needs into specific (SMART) design input requirements.

Examples of stakeholder needs are:

- intended use
- indications for use
- Marketing claims
- performance and safety requirements,
- physical characteristics,
- human factors

- biocompatibility & toxicity requirements
- compatibility requirements (accessories)
- packaging and labelling regulatory requirements of intended markets,
- sterility requirements,

The typical documents required when establishing design inputs include:

- The creation of a formal design description detailing the intended use, user requirements and design inputs. (Note: the design description must align with the design input requirements.)
- A design and development plan which provides an estimation of timelines, resources required, responsibilities, project risks and scope of the project.
- Initial risk assessment which contains the user, design and component risks to be mitigated.
- Design concepts and technology overview.
- Business case report addressing the market size and market opportunity.

NOTE: Design input requires are also a requirement of FDA 21 CFR Part 820.30(C) Design Input

Incomplete requirements can have a serious and costly effect on the design and ultimate success of a product. If essential design requirements are omitted in error or otherwise, the impact on quality or functionality may not be detected until validation. This presents an expensive problem that may not be easily rectified. If design requirements are missed, a redesign may be necessary before a design can be released to production, thus causing delays to the project. Furthermore, if modifications are required to tooling, or process equipment, timelines can be impacted greatly. However, the safety and quality of the product must be paramount. Keeping one eye on the user requirements and intended use of the product is an important factor in avoiding gross design requirement failings.

The purpose of design input is to create a set of requirements that are written in a technical manner with an engineering and scientific level of detail. The use of qualitative terms in a concept document is both appropriate and practical. This is often not the case for a document to be used as a basis for design. The language used in the creation of Design inputs also has a profound impact on the direction and scope of a product. If a concept document describes the product to be suitable for "outside use", then there will be requirements with regards to insulation, water ingress and operating temperatures and so on.

Design input requirements must be comprehensive. This may be quite difficult for manufacturers who are implementing a system of design controls for the first time. Design input requirements fall into three categories with most products having requirements within all three categories including:

(1) Functional requirements detailing the operation of the device.
(2) Performance requirements detailing the performance requirements or expectations of the device in relation to accuracy, speed of response times, battery life, device safety and reliability etc.
(3) Interface requirements specifying features of the device which are critical to compatibility with external systems such as the patient interface.

Design input is the starting point for product design. The requirements which form the design input establish a basis for performing subsequent design tasks and validating the design. Therefore, development of a solid foundation of requirements is the single most important design control activity.

Many medical device manufacturers have experience with the adverse effects that incomplete requirements can have on the design process. A frequent complaint of developers is that "there's never time to do it right, but there's always time to do it over." If essential requirements are not identified until validation, expensive redesign and rework may be necessary before a design can be released to production.

What is the scope of the design input requirements development process and how much detail must be provided? The scope is dependent upon the complexity of a device and the risk associated with its use. For most medical devices, numerous requirements encompassing functions, performance, safety, and regulatory concerns are implied by the application. These implied requirements should be explicitly stated, in engineering terms, in the design input requirements.

There are many cases when it is impractical to establish every functional and performance characteristic at the design input stage. But in most cases, the form of the requirement can be determined, and the requirement can be stated with a to-be-determined (TBD) numerical value or a range of possible values. This makes it possible for reviewers to assess whether the requirements completely characterize the intended use of the device, judge the impact of omissions, and track incomplete requirements to ensure resolution.

For complex designs, it is not uncommon for the design input stage to consume as much as thirty percent of the total project time. Unfortunately, some managers and developers have been trained to measure design progress in terms of hardware built, or lines of software code written. They fail to realize that building a solid foundation saves time during the implementation. Part of the solution is to structure the requirements documents and reviews such that tangible measures of progress are provided.

Design input requirements should be unambiguous. That is, each requirement should be able to be verified by an objective method of analysis, inspection, or testing. For example, it is insufficient to state that a catheter must be able to withstand repeated flexing. A better requirement would state that the catheter should be formed into a 50 mm diameter coil and straightened out for a total of fifty times with no evidence of cracking or deformity. A qualified reviewer could then make a judgment whether this specified test method is representative of the conditions of use.

Quantitative limits should be expressed with a measurement tolerance. For example, a diameter of 3.5 mm is an incomplete specification. If the diameter is specified as 3.500±0.005 mm, designers have a basis for determining how accurate the manufacturing processes have to be to produce compliant parts, and reviewers have a basis for determining whether the parts will be suitable for the intended use.

The set of design input requirements for a product should be self-consistent. It is not unusual for requirements to conflict with one another or with a referenced industry standard due to a simple oversight. Such conflicts should be resolved early in the development process. The environment in which the product is intended to be used should be properly characterized. For example, manufacturers frequently make the mistake of specifying "laboratory" conditions for devices which are intended for use in the home. Yet, even within a single country, relative humidity in a home may range from 20 percent to 100 percent (condensing) due to climactic and seasonal variations. Household temperatures in many climates routinely exceed 40 °C during the hot season. Altitudes may exceed 3,000 m, and the resultant low atmospheric pressure may

Design Outputs

The purpose of the design selection(output) phase is to provide a range of design options and solutions with the relevant evidence to show the effectiveness of the same. Often proof of concept (POC) or proof of principle (POP) trials may be used to verify effectiveness of solutions. POC/POP testing can involve making some limited prototypes. Any documents created in the previous phase, design input, should be reviewed and updated if required. There should be no contradictions or gaps between the documented inputs and outputs.

NOTE: Design outputs are also a requirement of FDA 21 CFR Part 820.30(D) Design Output

During this phase, product specifications (PS) and the device master record (DMR) are generated to define the design output. Planning for process validation and manufacturing begins during this phase often with the creation of a validation master plan (VMP). In any design office or factory setting, a lot of data and paperwork are generated. Therefore, it is important to be able to make the distinction between what is a design output and what is not. The first way of identifying a design output is to verify if it is listed as a task, a deliverable or listed in the design and development plan. If this is the case, then it is classified as a design output. Furthermore, if it describes or defines a design feature, it can also be classed as a design output.

The quality system requirements for design output can be separated into two elements: Design output should be expressed in terms that allow adequate assessment of conformance to design input requirements and should identify the characteristics of the design that are crucial to the safety and proper functioning of the device. This raises two fundamental issues for developers:

(1)What constitutes design output? AND (2) Are the form and content of the design output suitable? The first issue is important because the typical development project produces voluminous records, some of which may not be categorized as design output. On the other hand, design output must be reasonably comprehensive to be effective. As a general rule, an item is design output if it is a work product, or deliverable item, of a design task listed in the design and development plan, and the item defines, describes, or elaborates an element of the design implementation. Examples include block diagrams, flow charts, software high-level code, and system or subsystem design specifications. The design output in one stage is often part of the design input in subsequent stages. Design output includes production specifications as well as descriptive materials which define and characterize the design.

Design Review

Formal design reviews are critical to the efficacy of design control, and ultimately, the market success of the device. They should be planned for up front in the design development plan. Changes late in the design cycle are much more expensive than those made early on. Design reviews can play an important role in identifying changes in a timely manner and thus prevent costly redesigns close to the launch date. The FDA QSR clearly specifies the need for independent reviewers. Independent reviewers must be far enough removed from the design in order to provide an objective review.

NOTE: Design Review is required per FDA CFR Part 820.30(E) Design review

Design review should:
- provide feedback to designers on existing or emerging problems
- assess project progress
- provide confirmation that the project is ready to move on to the next phase of development

Many types of reviews occur during the course of developing a product. Reviews may have both an internal and external focus. Reviews are important in ensuring that the input requirements are not forgotten as the project progresses. Secondly, there must be "agreement" between the user requirements and design inputs versus the design outputs. A formal review of the design input requirements early in the development process is normally completed. The number of reviews depends upon the complexity of the device.

Many formal design reviews take the form of a meeting. At this meeting, the designer(s) may make presentations to explain the design implementation, and persons responsible for verification activities may present their findings to the reviewers. Reviewers may ask for clarification or additional information on any topic, and add their concerns to any raised by the presenters. This portion of the review is focused on finding problems, not resolving them. There are many approaches to conducting design review meetings. In simple cases, the technical assessor and reviewer may be the same person, often a project manager or engineering supervisor, and the review meeting is a simple affair in the manager's office. For more elaborate reviews, detailed written procedures are desirable to ensure that all pertinent topics are discussed, conclusions accurately recorded, and action items documented and tracked.

NOTE: Design Review is required per FDA 21 CFR CFR Part 820.30(f) Design Verification

Design Validation

Design validation is required for the product to ensure the device meets the user requirements and intended use. Above all, it ensures the device operates reliably and safely. Process validation is required in order to confirm manufacturing specifications and the Device Master Record (DMR). However, process validation is separate to design control and is covered in *Chapter 6 - Process Validation*.

NOTE: Design Validation required per 21 FDA CFR 820.30(G) Design Validation

Verification examines design outputs at the different phases of the process while design validation confirms that all user needs are achieved even when subject to anticipated sources of variation such as materials, processing equipment, suppliers and so on.

Validation Review

Validation may expose deficiencies in the original assumptions concerning user needs and intended uses. A formal review process should be used to resolve any such deficiencies.

As with verification, the perception of a deficiency might be judged insignificant or erroneous, or a corrective action may be required.

Many medical devices do not require clinical trials. However, all devices require clinical evaluation and should be tested in the actual or simulated use environment as a part of validation. This testing should involve devices which are manufactured using the same methods and procedures expected to be used for ongoing production. While testing is always a part of validation,
additional validation methods are often used in conjunction with testing, including analysis and inspection methods, compilation of relevant scientific literature, provision of historical evidence that similar designs and/or materials are clinically safe, and full clinical investigations or clinical trials.

Some manufacturers have historically used their best assembly workers or skilled lab technicians to fabricate test articles, but this practice can obscure problems in the manufacturing process. It may be beneficial to ask the best workers to evaluate and critique the manufacturing process by trying it out, but pilot production should simulate as closely as possible the actual manufacturing conditions.

Validation should also address product packaging and labelling. These components of the design may have significant human factors implications and may affect product performance in unexpected ways. For example, packaging materials have been known to cause electrostatic discharge (ESD) failures in electronic devices. If the unit under test is delivered to the test site in the test engineer's briefcase, the packaging problem may not become evident until after release to market. Validation should include simulation of the expected environmental conditions, such as temperature, humidity, shock and vibration, corrosive atmospheres, etc. For some classes of device, the environmental stresses encountered during shipment and installation far exceed those encountered during actual use and should be addressed during validation.

<u>Design Transfer</u>

The purpose of design transfer is to finalise all deliverables for filing with regulatory agencies. As the design output is finalised, the design is transferred into production specifications (drawings, manufacturing, test, and inspection procedures). Production specifications must ensure that manufactured devices are consistently and reliably produced within product and process capabilities, meeting all quality requirements.

Production and Service Provision

This section may not apply to all medical devices. However, devices that do require service and provision must have quality system elements that address (1) control of production and service provision – both general and specific requirements, (2) specific requirements for sterile medical devices, (3) validation of equipment and processes for production and service provision, (4) traceability and identification, (5) preservation of product controls with regard to monitoring and measuring medical devices.

Control of Monitoring and Measuring equipment

For processes involved in product realisation the manufacturer must identify what monitoring and measuring is required ensure the product or service meets the customer requirements. Calibration procedures, standards and records are requirement to demonstrate compliance.

Measurement Analysis

Sections

General requirements 8.1
Monitoring and measurement 8.2
Control of nonconforming products 8.3
Analysis of data 8.4
Improvement 8.5

General Requirements of measurement analysis requires appropriate measurement and inspection methods to be in place. Methods must be validation and equipment must be validated.

Monitoring and feedback depends on the gathering of data. Sources of data includes.

-Customer complaints
-Review of regulatory market surveillance
-Repair/servicing if applicable

Non-conforming product must be controlled and segregated to prevent use by the consumer or patient.

PART II Good Manufacturing Practices

Introduction

Good Manufacturing Practices are a set of practices that are required in order to comply with industry standards and regulations. GMP helps to minimise the risks involved during manufacturing and helps to ensure products meet quality and regulatory standards. A GMP quality system ensures that products are consistently produced and controlled according to predefined quality standards. It is designed to minimise the risks involved in any pharmaceutical production that cannot be eliminated through testing the final product.

Often, a broader term is used in industry -GxP-where the "x" is used as an umbrella letter representing different subjects or disciplines in industry. Some prime examples include GLP (Good Laboratory Practice), GDP (Good Documentation Practice), GEP (Good Engineering Practice) and GMP (Good Manufacturing Practices). Furthermore, the use of a lower case "c" as a prefix indicates "current" or "up-to-date". cGMP stands for "Current Good Manufacturing Practices. This means that some conventions or practices are subject to change within the industry. Therefore, it is important to be up-to-date in the application of cGxP or Cgmp. There are multiple regulators and organisations that provide definitions of "Good Manufacturing Practices". They include Organisations such as the World Health Organisation (WHO) and the International Society of Pharmaceutical Engineering (ISPE). Other definitions are offered by bodies such as the American competent authority for Food and Drug Administration. It is good to have an awareness of how organisations, bodies and competent authorities define GMP, and one should always review the "local" regulatory landscape. Below some definitions are provided to provide a feel for GMP and highlight the common thread between definitions.

W.H.O. World Health Organisation-"Good Manufacturing Practices (GMP, also referred to as 'cGMP' or 'current Good Manufacturing Practice') is the aspect of quality assurance that ensures that medicinal products are consistently produced and controlled to the quality standards appropriate to their intended use and as required by the product specification."

Food and Drug Administration: cGMP refers to the Current Good Manufacturing Practice regulations enforced by the US Food and Drug Administration (FDA). cGMPs ensure systems are properly designed and monitored, safeguarding the control of manufacturing processes and facilities. Adherence to the cGMP regulations ensures the identity, strength, quality, and purity of drug products by requiring that manufacturers of medications adequately control manufacturing operations. This includes establishing strong Quality Management Systems, obtaining appropriate quality raw materials, establishing robust operating procedures, detecting and investigating product quality deviations and maintaining reliable testing laboratories. This formal system of controls at a pharmaceutical company, if adequately put into practice, helps to prevent instances of contamination, mix-ups, deviations, failures and errors. This assures that drug products meet their quality standards.

MHRA (Medicines and Healthcare Products Regulatory Agency) defines GMP as follows:

"Good Manufacturing Practice (GMP) is that part of quality assurance which ensures that medicinal products are consistently produced and controlled to the quality standards appropriate to their intended use and as required by the marketing authorisation (MA) or product specification. GMP is concerned with both production and quality control. Many of the drivers of GMP in effect are also benefits to the manufacturer. Good manufacturing practices are an expected practice in regulated industries and a manufacturer must meet all relevant GMP regulations if they wish to manufacture within a country or sell to a particular market. It is important to maintain accurate, complete, up-to-date and consistent information to ensure patient safety and reduce any potential risks."

Documentation Creation

The principles of GDP should be applied at the document creation stage. As most people are familiar with softcopy or electronic documents, some of these points are obvious but nonetheless need to be made. All documents should be electronically written and not handwritten except for execution of protocols, test results and adding entries. Documents that are approved controlled should be:

Accurate and free from errors
Have revision or version controlled
Should have an effective date or date of release

Approval of Documents

Document approval must be completed by trained and appropriately experienced personnel. Often companies will use an approval matrix which explains which people are required to approve each document. For example, an EHS (Environment Health and Safety) officer would be required to approve a risk assessment.

Signatures

A signature on any document is legally binding so remember to read and understand what is being signed for. Every signature should also include the date in the correct format. If a signature appears within the same document alongside initials, substituting a full signature with initials and date is generally acceptable. This practice is common when large documents are being completed.

Date and Time Format

A standardised approach to dates and times is important especially within large global organisations. For instance, in the USA, the norm is to place the month before the date, whereas in Ireland and Great Britain it is common to write the day of the month followed by the month. Most companies would define their date and time format in an SOP or procedure.

The date and time format can also be configured in Word documents and Excel worksheets to align with a companies preferred date and time format.

Handwritten Entries

When a handwritten entry is required such as a signature or a test result, indelible ink must be used. Many companies will have an SOP or procedure that states the specific ink colour required. If an entry of a test result or test data isn't completed at the time of execution, this constitutes a late entry. Backdating an entry or signature is forbidden. Always use the correct and current date.

How Are Mistakes Corrected?

This is a critical area of GDP. Failure to follow the requirements of GDP when correcting mistakes is the most common failure when it comes to documentation in industry. The method of correcting mistakes using GDP allows for a person looking at the document for the first time to clearly see the original entry and the corrected entry. This maintains the integrity of the document. In order to identify the changes and corrections, certain rules must be followed. No overwriting is allowed and white-out or Tipp-Ex is not allowed.

Accuracy

Accuracy of information provided in documents is critical in the life science industry. As the end user is a patient, inaccurate records or documents could cause serious injury or death. Controlled documents are also legal documents and could be called upon if recalls, litigation or investigations arise.

Many documents used in the manufacture of medical devices are designed to record information or test results. These test results are then used to disposition (pass or fail) batches of product. Inaccurate information could risk the release and distribution of defective product. This has a potential impact on both the business and the patient or user.

Blank Spaces

On completion of a document such as a logbook or record, no blanks spaces should be left unfilled. This is to avoid late entries and also to prevent confusion. Blank spaces or blank fields should have a diagonal line drawn neatly across the space, the letters "N/A" written and the entry signed and dated. If the reason for "N/A" is not evident then it is wise to include an explanatory note or sentence.

Data Transcription

Transcribing is the process of transferring data from one source to another. This is often required when raw data is involved. When data is in raw format it may need to be entered into a Microsoft Excel sheet. When transcribing data remember that all original raw data must be stored in case it is needed at a future date. After the data is transcribed it must be verified by a second person to check for any errors or omissions.

Revision Control

Controlled documents should always have a version number or revision number electronically on each page of the document. This is similar to books which always list what edition they are e.g. first edition or second edition. Revision control is a key element of the Quality Management Systems in place in regulated industries. As the need for changes in the document arises, the controlled document can be amended/updated. With each update the version number revises also. Some companies will use alphabetic revision control and to a lesser extent numeric revision control (Version A, Version B or Version 01, Version 02).

Attachments

Attachments to controlled documents can include training records, data sheets, lab results and so on. It is important that attachments are identified for traceability purposes. If the attached becomes detached from the main document, the attachment should be identifiable. It is best practice to include a reference number on the attachment if available. If the attachment consists of several pages, each page should be numbered in Page X of Y format if not electronically done so. And remember, hand written entries must be accompanied by a signature and date. Always use staples to attach documents together. Glue or paper clips are not acceptable.

Document Lifecycle

GDP applies to all the different stages of a document's lifecycle. These stages include creation, review, approval, issuing, completion of records, revision, updating, retirement and storage. Storage a.k.a. retention is an important stage and often a legal requirement for medical devices and pharmaceutical products. For consumer OTC medicines a 5-year retention of quality records often suffices. For implants such as TKRs or Total Knee Replacements, a 90-year retention period is required. This ensures that traceability and a quality record is available if the need arises.

Test Results

This section provides an overview on the correct handling of test results. Test results can be generated from various types of product testing such as visual inspection, dimensional inspection and chemical analysis. The recording of all test results should be completed on an approved form. This is to ensure that the correct information is being recorded and the same approach is taken by different people who might have to complete testing.

Calculations

There are different ways calculations can be completed. Many simple calculations can be done by an individual using a calculator, alternatively, a software package such as Minitab or an Excel sheet can be used to complete complex calculations. It should be clear to the reader what calculation is required, what the formula is and how the calculation is completed.

If the formula used is not included on the sheet, it should be referenced in a controlled document. Care is also required when recording numbers of several decimal places in length, as rounding error can be introduced.

Units of Measurement

The most important thing to remember is consistency in units of measurement when recording data or making calculations. Consult your company procedure if available to determine the correct units of measurement. Many U.S. companies use imperial units e.g. inches, pounds etc. In Europe the International System of Units or SI is used, e.g. millimetres and kilograms.

What Is Quality?

Quality can be defined as the ability to consistently produce products meeting the same specifications time after time. Products must be safe, pure, uniform and effective. Specifications can be set down internally within a company, however, depending on the product, external specifications from regulators or standards may be required.

Patient safety is the primary focus of any pharmaceutical drug or medical device. This is the expectation of any patient or user. Secondly, the patient or user is interested in receiving an effective product. It is product specifications that ensure these criteria are accounted for.

What Is A Quality Management System?

A Quality Management System, often abbreviated to (QMS) is any system based on a collection of business processes that are primarily focused on providing safe and quality products that consistently meet customer requirements. The core themes of a QMS are outlined below.

Customer and Regulatory Focus

An understanding of the customer needs and requirements should be evident within the organisation and with the future vision of the company. The company should have an understanding of the regulatory landscape as this is subject to change over time. In turn the company should be positioned to respond to that change.

Leadership

To truly lead, one must be accepted in the hearts and minds of those they lead. Authentic leadership pays off. A leader should foster a sense of togetherness and common vision. A leader is anyone who influences or directs people either formally or informally. We are all leaders to some extent.

Involvement

Engagement by everyone across an organisation is now recognised as being key in the successful deployment of any Quality Management System. Everyone should have a voice within the company. As the saying goes "we are only as strong as the weakest link" is very apt.

Systems Management

This essentially means that systems are defined and described in writing along with the appropriate responses to expected issues that arise. Effective systems management must ensure that the various systems work in support of each other and communicate effectively with one another.

Decision Making

In order to make the right decision, the person empowered to make the decision must be informed. To be correctly informed one must have the correct details and facts available. In a manufacturing environment the facts are essentially data and the analysis of data. During manufacturing or processing, data is generated as a result of monitoring and measurement of products and the related processes.

Supplier Management

Don't ruffle your suppliers' feathers. Security of supply is key in delivering products to customers or patients again and again, Raw materials or sub-components sourced from external suppliers must always be sourced at the right price and time with the emphasis on getting the best quality possible.

Continuous Improvement

For IS0 13485 continuous improvement refers to improving the effectiveness of the Quality Management System. It is harder to drive improvement of the product due to regulatory and practical requirements. This is a key difference in contrast to ISO 19001:2008 as there is a requirement to continually improve both product and processes.

Quality Management Systems

The key elements of a QMS are listed below. The ISO Standard, ISO 9001, is a global Quality Management standard used by thousands of organisations and companies. This standard sets out the requirements of a QMS.

Quality Policy: A company will document their commitment and approach to quality within their organisation. It usually sets out how they plan to achieve a high and consistent standard of quality. It should in some way speak to the customer or end user.

Quality Objectives: Quality objectives can be documented in a Quality Plan at site or organisational level. An effective way of defining quality objectives is use of the SMART method. SMART stands for Specific, Measurable, Achievable, Realistic and Timely.

Quality Manual: An in-house guidance document to provide a framework for achieving the quality objectives.

Organisational Structure and Responsibilities: Organisational charts can be used to map out the company structure. Roles and responsibilities can be documented in site quality plans, job descriptions and Standard Operating Procedures.

Data Management: A coherent approach to the provision, storage and maintenance of data.

Processes: Processes are defined and documented.

Resources: Resources must be properly understood, allocated and linked across the organisation.

Product Quality & Customer Satisfaction: The proper management and investigation of complaints is important to reduce future instances from reoccurring. Continual engagement with the end user or customer is critical.

Continuous improvement including corrective and preventive action- where continuous improvement projects and initiatives are encouraged and supported. The application of a CAPA system to ensure quality is maintained and consistent.

Maintenance: A Preventative Maintenance schedule is in place and managed accordingly.

Sustainability: All work practices are sustainable and consistent throughout the lifecycle of processes and products.

Auditing: Systems are auditable and maintained to allow internal or external review and audit.

Engineering Change Control: Where changes are required to validated processes or equipment, changes are managed and introduced under change control.

A common acronym used to highlight the aims of Good Manufacturing Practices (GMP) is SPUE which stands for Safe-Pure-Uniform-Effective. This definition is particularly suited to pharmaceutical products as the chemicals and drugs used need to be pure and free of contaminants. Furthermore, they need to be uniform, meaning they will have the same constituents from tablet to tablet and batch to batch. A description of each word is shown below:

SAFE- the product has the right ingredients if it is a drug product. It is packaged as intended and correctly labelled in order to provide identification and safe use.

PURE- it is free of contaminants, foreign matter, chemicals and harmful microbes.

UNIFORM- The product is manufactured consistently and will have the same quality between batches manufactured on different days.

EFFECTIVE- Ultimately, the product must be effective in treating the medical condition. To be effective, it requires the correct ingredients, the correct amount of ingredients and correct packaging to maintain the product stability over time.

Quality Management

Quality: Degree to which a set of inherent properties of a product, system or process fulfils requirements.

Risk: defined as the combination of the probability of occurrence of harm and the severity of that harm.

Management: Systematic process for the assessment, control, communication and review of risks to the quality of the drug (medicinal) product across the product lifecycle. Achieving an effective product design, requires in depth knowledge of the customer requirements, clinical or medical need, regulatory requirements, and the manufacturing technology to be used. This collective knowledge or "knowledge space" ensures a robust and quality product is more likely to be designed that will meet the market requirements. Literature, engineering studies and the qualification and experience of employee's all contribute to the knowledge space. From this knowledge space, the most stable and effective design should be selected with product quality and safety as key factors. Furthermore, the quality of the product is then controlled and maintained within what can be described as the control space. During the design stage of product development, specifications are created to describe the attributes and features of the product. The output of the design stage is to have the required product specification documents available as inputs to equipment selection and process selection. Examples of some specifications include Raw material specifications, intermediate product specifications and finished product specifications. Specifications contain information on various features and product attributes such as dimensions, formulation, purity, cleanliness, surface finish and so on. The critical requirements stated in specification are often referred to as Critical Quality Attributes (CQAs) and Critical Process Parameters (CPPs)

Critical Quality Attributes (CQA): a particular property of a material, product or output of a process that is key to the product performance and safety.

Critical Process Parameters (CPP): a process parameter such as temperature or time that when varied it impact the quality or CQA of a product.

What Is RFT?

Right First Time strives to create a culture of excellence. People are challenged with performing their tasks always in the correct manner to achieve the correct results always - *right the first time*. RFT is the enabler to providing customers worldwide with accessible, high quality and advanced healthcare solutions which comply with cGMP requirements.

What is 5S?

5S is a Japanese methodology of organising and storing items in a work or lab environment. It has been adopted by many Western companies as a tool to help maintain standards and reduce errors and mix-ups. The "5s" represents each stage of the method.

Sort

Sorting out any items that are not in use and removing to a more appropriate area or to storage or the bin.

Set-in-Order

The idea of "Set-in-Order" is to be always organised. "A place for everything and everything in its place. "If we "set-in-order" we can help to make live processing and testing more efficient and reduce the risk of errors, omissions and accidents.

Shine

Regular cleaning is an important practice and it is always helpful to "Clean as you go."

Standardise

Implement standard practices through SOPs and training. Standardisation can also be applied to work station layout.

Sustain

Make it a habit! After implementing a 5s methodology, it is only effective if continuous efforts are made to "sustain" the changes.

PART 3 Validation

Introduction

Validation planning plays a key role in the qualification and validation of new equipment and processes. It also has a role in established processes and is used to plan and manage the ongoing validation requirements within a company. So why the need for validation plans? Firstly, the requirement for validation within medical device and pharmaceutical companies is a legal and regulatory one. The Food and Drug Administration (FDA) stipulates validation as a regulatory requirement of Good Manufacturing Practices (GMP) for both pharmaceuticals (21 CFR 211) and medical devices (21 CFR 820). Validation plans act like a qualification plan that can be used to document strategies, technical rationales and key deliverables. They are a regulatory requirement for medicinal products manufactured in the United States and Europe.

Although not stated in 21 CFR Part 820 (Medical Devices), validation planning is an important activity that helps to document the validation strategy and is commonplace with medical device manufacturers. In Europe, EudraLex (V4 GMP) is the collection of rules and regulations governing medicinal products in the European Union which also require validation planning.

All equipment, processes, facilities and utilities that are GxP impacting need to be qualified. To facilitate the validation efforts, a Validation Plan (VP) creates a roadmap and structure to meet the validation requirements. For simple processes or simple equipment qualifications, a stand-alone validation plan may not be required and can be captured within a protocol or change control. The requirements of validation plans can be driven by a procedure which may be local to a site or factory or may be corporate and applicable to multiple sites. Consistency of requirements can also be managed by the use of an approved validation plan template.

Apart from regulatory or procedural requirements to create a validation plan, there are many other beneficial reasons to complete one. A validation plan acts as a top level document that can pull together the many references, protocols, reports and rationales that make up a project. It is also a powerful asset to introduce new staff and team members to a project or process who need to get up to speed quickly and comprehensively. Validation plans are often the first documents an auditor will request to see in relation to a new process or new product introduction. They force the various stakeholders to sit down and agree upon the strategy and any technical rationales required to deliver a successful project.

Validation Plans

Validation plans can be divided into three different types or configurations. Depending on the validation activity or the project, a validation plan may take the form of a (1) Site Validation Plan (aka Site Master Validation Plan) (2) Master Validation Plans (MVPs) or (3) Individual Validation Plans (VPs).

From the outset, it is important to highlight that different companies may adopt different terminology with regard to validation planning. Typically, large companies will have a site validation plan aka site master validation plan or equivalent document.

A site MVP details the products, processes and associated validation protocols and reports for a manufacturing site/factory. It is the overarching validation plan. Typical components of a site MVP include: description of products and processes, test methods (analytical, physical), specifications, an up-to-date list of utility qualifications, equipment qualifications and process validations.

An MVP encompasses all aspects of a validation strategy and may include multiple processes, multiple pieces of equipment/machines that require validation. MVPs are common for new product introductions. Although not stated in 21 CFR Part 820, MVPs are useful in documenting the validation status.

An individual validation plan generally details the validation strategy of one piece of equipment or machine, therefore, an individual validation plan tends to be limited to a handful of pages.

Nonetheless, it is valuable in documenting the validation approach and is a central document that can detail process development reports, specifications and so on.

Bracketing

A family or matrix approach to validation can be used where similar products are produced using the same equipment and processes. A particular product size or product configuration may be selected to represent the "worst-case" product. Therefore, by qualifying the worst case, all of the other products within the family are considered validated. Matrix or family approaches must be clearly documented with technical rationale provided in advance of any qualification activities. This can be addressed in a validation plan or within a protocol. Alternatively, a technical report or product development report can be created and referenced. Taking a family of products, the worst case product might be, the smallest, the largest, the heaviest, or the product requiring the greatest precision and so on.

Changes to the Validated State

Revalidation may be necessary under the following conditions:

- change(s) in the actual process that may affect quality or its validation status
- change(s) in the product design which affects the process
- transfer of processes from one facility to another
- change of the application of the process
- change in materials
- change in a manufacturing agent (cleaning agent, oils, greases, coolant, detergents etc.)

The need for revalidation should be evaluated and documented. Evaluation needs to consider historical results from quality indicators, product changes, process changes, changes in external requirements (regulations or standards) and other such circumstances, as applicable. Revalidation may not be as extensive as the initial validation if the situation does not require that all aspects of the original validation be repeated.

Equipment and Software Validation

Introduction

Validation is *"Establishing documented evidence that provides a high degree of assurance that a specific process will consistently produce a product meeting its pre-determined specifications and quality attributes"*.

Equipment Qualification is to ensure that equipment is fit for its intended use. Therefore, equipment is validated to confirm it functions as intended and meets all requirements to manufacture product safely and consistently. FDA requires that "Each manufacturer shall ensure that all equipment used in the manufacturing process meets specified requirements and is appropriately designed, constructed, placed and installed to facilitate maintenance, adjustment, cleaning and use". In other words all manufacturing equipment, support facilities, measuring and test equipment must be "qualified". (FDA 21 CFR 820.70 (G))

Equipment qualification protocols are developed to document this testing and hence provide evidence on the functionality and consistency of the equipment. There are two distinct parts within the scope of equipment qualification, installation qualification and operational qualification. Often these subparts are abbreviated to IQ and OQ. Other combinations such as IOQE and IQ/OQ can be encountered within industry. This is often defined in a company's procedure or SOP relating to equipment validation.

Installation Qualification

We have previously defined Equipment Qualification (EQ) and the two components to it (IQ and OQ) as "Establishing by documented evidence that all key aspects of the equipment installation meets the manufacturer's specification"). IQ is required in order to ensure that the equipment is installed, positioned and sited in a manner that is safe and in-line with manufacturer's recommendations. Once a piece of equipment is sited, it must be integrated into the utilities that are required to operate the equipment. An example of typical checks is listed on the following page.

Operational Qualification

The second element of equipment qualification now must be considered; equipment-operational qualification. This is "Establishing by documented evidence that the equipment operates per specifications and over the required ranges and to required tolerances". Equipment is also tested to ensure alarms and controls operate as required and intended. Some typical checks included in an equipment-operational qualification are testing of alarms, control system testing, utility failures and functional and operational testing.

Types of Validation

With most equipment, systems and processes it is best practice to complete all qualification and validation activities in advance of the manufacture of any products for sale, commercial use and use in certain trials. The FDA provides clear definitions on the four types of validation which are explained below.

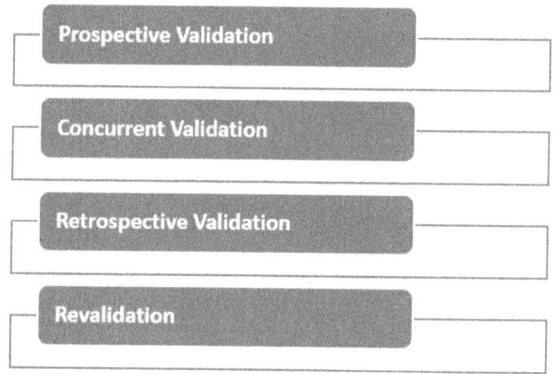

Prospective Validation

Establishing documented evidence **in advance** of process implementation that a process or system operates as intended. This is the preferred approach and is most common when new products must be validated before commercial manufacturing.

Concurrent Validation

Establishing documented evidence that a process operates as intended, based on information generated during process implementation. Concurrent means that the outputs and performance of the system are monitored at the time of manufacturing which can include commercial lots.

Retrospective Validation

Retrospective validation is used for facilities or processes that have not completed formal validation. Historical data or a retrospective review can provide the evidence that the process or facility is operated as intended. This type of validation is uncommon.

Revalidation involves the re-execution of validation activities in order to maintain a validated state. This can be a result of substantial changes to product attributes, specification or changes to the manufacturing process itself. Other reasons a partial or full revalidation may be required involve instances where product quality issues have increased.

Software Validation

Where there is potential to affect product conformance to requirements or where software or IT systems provide support to aspects of quality management, validation is required.

Most companies categorise software validations to account for the different applications of software and IT systems. For example, enterprise systems, such as the drawing package SolidWorks, would be validated in a different manner to manufacturing systems that contain software (a.k.a. embedded software).

"Embedded" software is where the software is integrated into the manufacturing equipment. Embedded software is typically validated during the equipment qualification stage, process validation stage or test method validation. Enterprise software falls outside of equipment or process validation but does require validation if it impacts product quality or is used to make quality decisions. Standalone systems such as ERP (Enterprise Resource Planning) systems also require validation.

Software Validation and GAMP

Good Automated Manufacturing Practice (GAMP) is a set of guidelines for manufacturers and users of automated systems in regulated industries. These guidelines are particularly important for the medical device, pharmaceutical and biopharmaceutical industries. The application of GAMP and validation of automated systems in manufacturing helps ensure that regulated medical devices and medicinal products have the required quality and are manufactured according to good practices, meet regulatory and legal requirements and ensure patient safety. GAMP ensures quality is in-built into each stage of the manufacturing process. Therefore, GAMP has a place in all aspects of automation and production, including the handling of raw materials, control of facilities and equipment etc.

Automated System: Term used to cover a broad range of systems, including automated manufacturing equipment, control systems, automated laboratory systems, manufacturing execution systems and computers running laboratory or manufacturing database systems. The automated system consists of the hardware, software and network components, together with the controlled functions and associated documentation. Automated systems are sometimes referred to as computerised systems.

Commercial Off-the-Shelf (COTS): Configurable programs and stock programs that can be configured to specific user applications by "filling in the blanks", without (COTS) altering the basic program.

Computer System Validation: A process that confirms by examination and provision of objective evidence that the computer system conforms to user needs and intended uses. System validation is a process for achieving and maintaining compliance with GxP regulations and fitness for intended use by adoption of life cycle activities, deliverables, and controls.

GAMP 5: Is a set of guidelines that offers a risk-based approach to ensuring the compliance of GxP-impacting computerised systems.

V- Model: Is a development process which sets out a roadmap of stages and deliverables during a project.

21 CFR Part 820: FDA requirements pertaining to medical devices.

User Requirement Specification, URS: The URS is a critical document that defines the requirements of the computerised system and agreement to the requirements.

Software Requirement Specification, SRS: An SRS can be written to interpret the requirements of a URS and how they relate to the requirement or how the requirement is met in practical terms regarding software.

Functional Design Specification, FDS: A functional design specification is a document that specifies how particular requirements are met – this can be a combination of how the equipment/process operates mechanically/automatically etc. An FDS is typically written in response to a URS.

Computer System Validation Life Cycle

The Computer System Validation Life Cycle refers to all activities from initial concept to retirement of a computer system. The life cycle of the system includes the defining of, and performance of activities in a systematic way from conception, requirements, development or configuration, testing, release and operational use. The four GAMP life cycle phases include:

- Concept
- Planning and project stage
- Operation
- Retirement

The concept stage is concerned with understanding the need or the problem to be addressed. We will see that the User Requirement Specification (along with other specifications) and the initial risk assessment help to drive a project forward in a systematic manner. The most common life cycle approach for computerised and automated systems is the V-Model. The GAMP based V-model lays out a roadmap which facilitates the validation of equipment and automated systems.

The planning and project stage involves the planning of the validation effort required to implement the system into the business area(s) based on identification and approval of system concept. This phase includes assessments of the regulatory and system risks, supplier assessment, development of validation strategies, identification of deliverables that will be generated, definition of the business process the system will support as well as the user requirements which the system will fulfil. Design, development and configuration of the hardware and software are also required to meet the system requirements as per specifications. In case of custom software components, this effort could also include detailed software design and developmental testing to ensure readiness for verification testing.

The verification stage confirms that specifications have been met and releases the system for use. This phase will involve multiple stages of reviews and testing depending on the system type, the development method applied and its use. Once verification activities have begun any changes to the system must be captured through change control. On successful completion of the verification activities, the system is then released for effective use. The test strategy and other verification activities will vary widely between simple equipment and more complex customised/configurable systems. The verification and validation approach is typically agreed and detailed in the validation planning stage. The VP can be updated accordingly as the project develops with more detail being added. Alternatively, a test strategy document or matrix could be written to provide more specific test plans.

Validation reporting requirements vary depending upon the scope of the system and should also be driven by a procedure and template. The validation plan can also outline the deliverables and what needs to be addressed in the report. A Validation Summary Report (VSR) must be written which summarises the results of executing the VP. The documents created for the validation activities summarise (or point to summaries) of the testing performed. Finally, the VSR indicates the acceptance of the system/equipment by the user and by the project team stating that the equipment is released for commercial operation/production.

The operation phase supports the need to maintain compliance and fitness for intended use after the system is released for normal use. It is important to ensure the system remains within a continued validated state. All proposed or necessary changes to the system must be assessed and controlled as part of a change control process. Once the system has been accepted and released for use, the operation phase begins. This phase consists of maintaining the system's compliant state and fitness for intended use through the control of the procedures supporting the system's operational use.

During the operation phase the below activities are typically completed:

- Ongoing training
- Preventative maintenance
- Service management and performance monitoring
- Change control
- Periodic review
- Maintaining system security
- Records management
- Calibration

The retirement phase involves the planning and proper management of activities relating to the removal of systems from service (shutdown). The retirement should take into account the storage of any data and any data migration that needs to occur prior to retirement. The retirement plan, if needed, will outline the retirement strategy from the roles and activities that will be conducted to the removal of the system for use. A Retirement Summary Report is produced that documents the results of the activities defined in the retirement plan including:

- Retirement Plan and timelines.
- Summaries of any data migration activities.
- Identification of the storage location of documentation relating to the system.
- Obsoleting of SOPs.

It must be stressed that GAMP is a set of principles, a set of guidelines that aims to achieve compliant computerised systems that are fit for intended use. GAMP Guidelines differ to 21 CFR QSR regulations as they are not legal or statutory requirements. However, they represent industry best practice and compliment the validation efforts that are legal requirements and statutory requirements.

Regulatory Review

Software validation is a requirement of the quality system regulation, 21 Code of Federal Regulations (CFR) Part 820. Validation requirements apply to:

(1) software used as components in medical devices
(2) software that is itself a medical device
(3) software used in production of the device or in implementation of the device manufacturer's quality system.

Note: EU GMP Annex 11, provides information on the inspection of 'computerised systems'.

In addition, computer systems used to create, modify, and maintain electronic records and to manage electronic signatures are also subject to the validation requirements. Such computer systems must be validated to ensure accuracy, reliability, consistent intended performance and the ability to discern invalid or altered records. The regulated user should be able to demonstrate through the validation evidence that they have a high level of confidence in the integrity of both the processes executed within the controlling computer system and in those processes controlled by the computer system within the prescribed operating environment.

System Categorisation

GAMP 5 makes provision for four categories of software in order to distinguish the level of customisation/configurability that exists across software serving different functions.

> GAMP Software Category 1, Operating systems
> GAMP Software Category 2, Non-configured software
> GAMP Software Category 4, Configurable software packages
> GAMP Software Category 5, Custom software

GAMP Software Category 1, Operating Systems

Category 1, operating systems, covers established, commercially available operating systems.

These are not subject to validation themselves; the name and version of the operating system must, however, be documented and verified during Installation Qualification (IQ). Application software hosted on operating systems need to be validated.

GAMP Software Category 2, Non-configured Software

Category 3 covers commercially available, standard software packages and "off-the-shelf" solutions for certain processes. The configuration of the software packages should be limited to adaptation to the runtime environment (for example network and printer connections) and the configuration of the process parameters. The name and version of the standard software package should be documented and verified in an Installation Qualification (IQ). Special user requirements, such as security, alarms, messages, or algorithms must be documented and verified in an Operational Qualification (OQ).

GAMP Software Category 4, Configurable Software Packages

GAMP Software Category 4, Configurable Software Packages Category 4 covers configurable software packages that allow special business and manufacturing processes. This involves configuring predefined software modules. These software packages should only be considered as belonging to Category 4 if they are well-known and mature. Normally, a supplier audit is necessary. If this is not available, the software packages should be handled as Category 5. The name, version, and configuration should be documented and verified in an Installation Qualification (IQ). The functions of the software packages should be verified in terms of the user requirements in an Operational Qualification (OQ). The validation plan should take into account the life cycle model and an assessment of suppliers and software packages.

GAMP Software Category 5, Custom Software

GAMP Software Category 5, Custom Software Custom/Bespoke Software (GAMP Software Cat 5) is software that contains custom code designed or modified specifically for a particular customer. As the code is custom it presents a greater risk. This risk must be mitigated with the right approach to the validation.

GAMP Considerations

Correctly assigning a GAMP software category to equipment, a system or process is an important activity that should be completed early on in the planning stage of a project. There must be some degree of familiarity with the equipment or system. The manufacturer or vendor can be a source of information that may help the designation. In many cases, companies create tools or processes that help determine what GAMP software category applies. These have different names such as questionnaires, screening tools, planning tools etc.

Risk Assessments

A risk assessment process should be applied to cGxP computerised systems in order to identify and mitigate potential risks to (1) patient safety, (2) product quality and (3) data integrity. Results identified through a risk assessment help to determine the validation strategy, the effort and time required, and allow better targeting of the validation activities to the highest risks.

The Risk Assessment should be revised during the Software Development Life cycle (SDLC) if the functionality, requirements or intended use of the system changes. The risk assessment activity should also be evaluated during system build-up as well as when implementing changes. Risk assessment tools for cGxP computerised systems are typically completed during the planning stage, specification stage and post qualification if a change or update is required.

Planning Stage

Initial Impact/Risk Assessment – during the planning phase to identify the level of impact and GxP relevance of the system/equipment. (Tools used: High-Level Risk Assessment).

Specification Stage

Functional or Quality Risk Assessment – during the specification phase – identify potential risks and possible mitigations to be to be introduced to the process. (Tools used: Quality Risk Matrix, (p)FMEA).

Changes to the System

Impact Assessment of Changes – as part of the change control process in the system operational phase. The following diagram defines the risk assessment steps within the system life cycle (Tools used: Impact Assessment Checklist, Change Control Procedures).

Traceability

A Traceability Matrix should be prepared as required in accordance with company and internal policy. It is also recommended by GAMP guidelines, ASTM E2500 and ISPE risk-based approach to validation. The matrix links the user requirements and specifications to the testing and validation activities. A traceability matrix illustrates that all user requirements are traceable to the verification/validation activity or vendor documents as relevant (FDS if applicable, design specifications etc.). Generally, individual organisations will have an approved template to work from. However, the URS structure can form the basis of the template, with additional columns added to document the test/verification method, reference documents (such as FDS and vendor specifications and design documents)

General Requirements

Configuration Identification

Software and hardware packages should be identified by a unique product identifier and a version number. For the software end-user, the parts of an automated system that are subject to configuration management should be clearly identified. The system should therefore be broken down into configuration items. These should be identified at an early phase of development so that a complete list of configuration items is defined and maintained. The application-specific items should have a unique name or version ID. The depth of detail when specifying the elements is decided by the needs of the system, and the organisation developing that system.

Requirements for the User ID and Password

User ID: The user ID of a system should have a minimum length agreed with the customer and should be unique within the system.

Password: A password should always consist of a combination of numeric and alphanumeric characters. When setting up passwords, the number of characters and a period after which a password expires should be stipulated. The structure of the password is normally selected to suit the specific customer. The configuration is described in the section ***Security Settings of Password Policy***.

Criteria for the structure of a password are as follows:
- Minimum length of the password
- Use of numeric and alphanumeric characters
- Case sensitivity

Audit Trail

The audit trail is a control mechanism of a system that allows all data entered or modified to be traced back to the original data. A reliable and secure audit trail is particularly important in conjunction with the creation, change or deletion of GMP relevant electronic records. In this case, the audit trail must archive and document all the changes or actions made along with the date and time. Typical contents of an audit trail must be recorded and describe the procedures "who changed what and when" (old value/new value).

Software Source Code Review

For GAMP Software Categories 4 and 5, source code review is advised unless the supplier has evidence of the same available for review. As part of Good Automated Manufacturing Practices, reviews should be completed as part of the development life cycle. If a source code review is not completed a justifiable rationale should be documented in an applicable document such as a validation master plan.

Deviations

A deviation can be simply described as an unintended event which causes a test or verification to fail to meet expected acceptance criteria. Each company or organisation should have a procedure detailing the management of deviations. It is critical that all deviations are identified, investigated and evaluated for their impact on product quality, the risk/impact to the patient and the impact on the qualification or validation. The basic components to a deviation are listed below:

- Deviation Description - provides the page and section of the deviation and an overall description e.g. document generation error, operator error, machine crash etc.

- Potential impact on product – does the deviation impact the product?

- Potential impact on validation/qualification – will the validation have to be repeated in part or in full?

- Investigation – DMAIC, RCA, fishbone diagram, 5Ws

- Root Cause- what is the concluding root cause?

- Planned Resolution- what actions are required to be implemented?

- Deviation Resolution (Actions completed) – were all the actions in the planned resolution implemented? What is the final result? Have the actions been effective?

Requalification

Over the lifetime of a piece of equipment, the need to requalify may arise. Therefore, any proposed change to equipment or a process must be assessed to see if the validated state will be impacted. It is therefore critical to understand clearly the nature of the change(s). Some scenarios where requalification of equipment may be required include:

- Major equipment repairs

- Moving equipment

- Changes to the upper and lower operating limits of the equipment

- Upgrading of software

- Hardware upgrades or changes

- Changes in performance and/or defect levels

After assessing any proposed changes based on the reasons listed above, a determination of the level of requalification is required. This may be limited to a partial requalification (addendum) or it may require a full requalification.

Process Validation

This chapter provides an introduction to process validation for medical devices. Process validation is a statutory and regulatory requirement for the manufacture of medical devices. Per FDA 21 Code of Federal Regulations process validation is a regulatory requirement of Good Manufacturing Practices (GMP) for both pharmaceuticals (21 CFR 211) and medical devices (21 CFR 820). In addition to the regulatory drivers, process validation is a requirement in order to obtain certification to international standards issued by many notified bodies. (E.g. ISO 13485 Medical Devices – Quality Management Systems, ASTM E2500- Standard Guide for Specification, Design, and Verification of Pharmaceutical and Biopharmaceutical Manufacturing Systems and Equipment etc.)

Traditional and New Approaches to Validation

Historically, process validation involved the testing and verification of all aspects of a process. While this may seem appropriate, it must be understood that in order to test/verify all aspects of a process, and for it to hold weight, this activity must be documented and recorded. In this respect, an "all aspects" approach to process validation can be burdensome to resources. The traditional approach largely used the V-Model which set out a sequence of deliverables that should be completed. The use of risk assessments were limited as all requirements of a system were tested and qualified.

In recent years, a risk-based approach has been increasingly endorsed by regulatory authorities and hence adopted by medical device manufacturers. One such standard is the ASTM E2500. As the title suggests, it is primarily used within pharmaceutical and biopharmaceutical industries; its principles and core approach can be adopted by medical device manufacturers also. ASTM E2500 was designed to make the implementation process for GMP systems and validation more cost-effective. It aims to achieve this based on scientific and risk-based principles, focusing on the risk to the patient. However, at just a five-page document, ASTM E2500 lacks the detail required in order to meet regulatory expectations. While different terminology and philosophies exist, they do not change the regulatory expectations relating to validation.

Both approaches exhibit common elements which include:

- ➢ Good engineering practices
- ➢ Planning
- ➢ Requirements definition (URS etc.)
- ➢ Design review
- ➢ Change management
- ➢ Documented testing and inspection

While many manufacturers may predominantly choose a particular approach, it is common to see elements of both approaches (traditional and risk based). Each individual company will shape its internal validation procedures to best suit the business needs of the company.

What Is Process-Operational Qualification (OQ-P)?

The ability of a process to produce product in accordance with pre-determined specifications under worst case conditions. PQ is only required if no worst-case conditions are evident.

What Is Process-Performance Qualification (PQ)?

www.ingramcontent.com/pod-product-compliance
Lightning Source LLC
Chambersburg PA
CBHW070305220526
4546SCB00004B/1749

The ability of a process to consistently produce product in accordance with predetermined specifications under anticipated conditions (normal/routine conditions). Before considering process validation in further detail, it is important to look at the prerequisites and other supporting activities required. These are examined in the sections below.

Stages of Process Validation

The three stages of process validation include:
- Process Design
- Process Validation
- Continued Process Monitoring

The commercial manufacturing process must be established during the process design phase. Some typical activities include:
- Definition of process inputs
- Effects of inputs
- Process outputs – CQAs (critical quality attributes)
- Establishing process windows
- DFMEA /PFMEA (design/process)

Design Control procedures should be developed to allow proper management of the process design stage. At the process design stage, the business must define the manufacturing process. This often involves liaising with vendors and Subject Matter Experts (SMEs). The process qualification stage looks at the validation of process design to confirm process is operating as intended and is capable of consistently producing product to meet quality requirements. Finally, stage 3, Continued Process Verification provides ongoing assurance through regular testing and verification to ensure the process is in control. Stage 3 is often referred to as In-Process Control or In-Process Testing (IPC/IPT). This data provides feedback to engineers allowing them to trend the performance of output data. This can identify deficient equipment, changes in wear tooling etc.

Fundamentals of Process Validation

The most important point when it comes to validation is that validation is neither exploratory nor investigative. Equally, it is not an engineering study. If you are ready to validate a system or process, all of the groundwork must be completed. This means critical parameters must be defined and documented, with technical rationale on why such parameters are critical etc. This body of work is typically done during a process development study or protocol. Process validation is confirming that a process is capable of consistently manufacturing product under anticipated conditions. Remember, validation should be representative of the commercial process, so any issues in process validation will be repeated in commercial manufacturing.

Consistency, a core principle of process validation, is typically demonstrated by producing three batches/runs for a Process Performance Qualification (PPQ). These batches should be representative of normal production i.e. the size of the batch should be typical of commercial volumes. The PQ study should be executed at nominal conditions, (often termed "anticipated conditions") essentially referring to a controlled environment. Controlled material and controlled parameters (CPPs) are required. Nominal settings should be selected for PQ.

Process Operational Qualification (OQ-P)

During the Operational Qualification-Process (OQ-P) study,

worst-case process conditions are normally employed. This may be worst case temperatures, speeds, feeds etc. The OQ-P should challenge the manufacture/processing of product at the limits of the processing window. If no worst-case conditions exist, then an OQ may not be required and only a performance qualification is required. A family or matrix approach is often used where similar products are to be validated. A particular product size or product configuration may be selected to represent the worst-case product. Therefore, by qualifying the worst case, all other products within that family of products would be considered validated. However, this approach must be clearly documented and technical rationale provided in advance of any qualification activities. This can be addressed in a validation plan or within a protocol.

Protocol Approval Check list

The validation protocol is the means in which objective evidence is documented and gathered. The validation protocol is therefore a critical document. It should clearly set out the approach to the validation, detailing methods, tests and verifications to be completed and the acceptance criteria that applies to such tests and verifications. Remember, a validation document is a legal and regulatory document and can be subject to detailed scrutiny. Below are some suggested general checks to apply when writing validation protocols.

Author:
- SOP available - Protocol conforms to validation procedure.
 - Ensure item numbers and batch size are correct.
 -Test methods are correct.

SME Reviewer:
- Is the protocol number correct?
-Review content of protocol for accuracy and completeness.
- Protocol conforms to validation procedures.

- Procedure and evaluation table are appropriate and correct.

Engineering:
- Review content of protocol for accuracy and completeness.
- Specifications and operating parameters are correct.

QC / Laboratory:
- Review content of protocol.
- Raw material specifications are in place.
- Finished product specifications are in place.
- Testing and sample size is correct.

Quality:
- Review content of protocol.
- Protocol conforms to SOPs.
- Evaluation and acceptance criteria are appropriate.

Process Performance Qualification

The purpose of the PPQ is to demonstrate the capability of the process to consistently manufacture product to pre-determined specifications under normal operating conditions and defined parameters.

Key principles of Process Performance Qualification

Validation is confirmation, so process validation is confirming that a process is capable of consistently manufacturing product under anticipated conditions.

- Lots should be produced consecutively (in sequence)

- Lots must meet the acceptance criteria set out in the protocol

- The lot size should be reflective of the intended lot size and also take into account normal variation

- If a family approach or matrix approach is used, the product selection must be clearly justified and documented

- Execute under anticipated conditions; essentially this refers to a controlled environment. Controlled material, controlled parameters (CPPs)

- Nominal settings should be selected for PPQ

Yield Data (aka Process Yield Data)

Process yield is a term used in manufacturing to represent the overall process performance. Yield is most often expressed as a percentage of goods/passing products. It reports the percentage of compliant units, that is units or products that meet the product acceptance criteria (e.g. CQAs). The remaining "bad" units are classified as defects or scrap. In some manufacturing processes, rework is possible or permitted.

Yield data often forms part of the acceptance criteria for a validation. The overall process yield for each batch should be calculated and compared to the starting process weights or units to determine loss due to processing as it is common to lose material during processing.

Continued Process Verification

Once the initial validation is completed it is important that the system or process remains within the validated state, meaning that the system remains in a state of controlling process systems that capture information and data about the performance of the process. The use of statistical trending techniques should be considered. Data analysis of process and product should also include trending of raw materials, components and finished product. The purpose of process monitoring is to ensure critical parameters remain within control limits. It also helps to identify increasing variability or instability within the process which can then be investigated. All processes must have an upper and lower limit. If a process parameter only has a one-sided limit, then provide rationale in the OQ protocol to justify why a one-sided parameter window is acceptable. This requirement is not applicable to parameters that are set points.

Revalidation (or Maintaining a Validated State)

Revalidation is sometimes required if the original validation is no longer valid or representative of the process. Some instances where revalidation must be considered include changes to the process that can affect the product quality or efficacy, a removal, or the addition of a processing step or transfer of the equipment to a different location. In many companies an impact assessment is conducted if there is a proposal to modify a manufacturing process. Some changes may not require any validation while others may require a verification run. When changes are proposed to the validated state of a process, the proposed changes must be fully understood in terms of the impact to product quality and the validated state. A risk assessment should be conducted to determine risks and appropriate mitigations.

Requalification

During the lifetime of a process or piece of equipment, the need to re-qualify may arise. Such need should be assessed according to a validation procedure. Generally, the same tools used in the original validation can be re-applied to identify the need to re-qualify and indicate what requirements must be included.

The first step must be a review of the existing qualification, as changes may not impact the validated state, or may only require a limited requalification. For example, moving a piece of equipment may only require requalification of the utilities such as compressed air or process water if the operation of the equipment is not impacted by the movement and re-siting. Some examples where re-qualification may be required include:

- Transferring a process from one plant to another plant
- Changes to the process settings which may impact the product quality
- Changes to the design of the product
- Changes to manufacturing aids (e.g. cleaning agents, jigs and fixtures)

Packaging Validation

This section outlines six key stages of the packaging validation life cycle. In order to describe the packaging life cycle in a structured and manageable format, the process can be sub-divided into 6 stages. It must be noted that an individual company will have its own interpretation of the required stages with different terminology or specific requirements. However, the intent of any approach should broadly align.

Stage 1 - Design and Development of Packaging
Stage 2 – Material(s), Equipment and Process Technology
Stage 3 - Material Performance and Suitability Testing
Stage 4 - Stability Testing
Stage 5 - Packaging Performance Testing
Stage 6 – Packaging Validation

Blister packing is a process whe pre-formed plastic packaging (blisters) manufactured using a cavity of a defined shape and size are used to pack a range of items including various personal tech-ware goods, foods, pharmaceuticals and medical devices. The primary component of a blister pack is a cavity or pocket which is made by forcing a material, usually a plastic into the cavity under vacuum and at deformation temperature. The resulting blister is often closed with cardboard, paperboard, foil or plastic depending on the product. The combination of the blister and lid or lidstock helps to protect products from the environment such as microbial contamination, humidity and foreign matter.

Most blisters made from plastics will provide good protection to the inner product. Often, it is the lid or lidstock that is the weaker of the two. Some lid materials are prone to tearing or puncturing and degradation over time. In addition, the area where the lid is bonded to the blister is a point of interest and must be inspected adequately to ensure a proper seal integrity is achieved. Not only is the movement of the product and force of the product a risk factor in damaging the package, but equally the design of the system should also account for handling and a degree of inappropriate handing as a safety factor.

Some manufacturers offer breathable-type seals which reduce the risk of condensation forming on the inside of the pack due to temperature and humidity differences that can occur during shipping or storage.

Stage 1 - Design and Development of Packaging

The design of medical packaging is equally as important as the products they contain. They ensure products are kept clean, sterile (if applicable) and essentially make them safe and effective when used. They need to serve the requirements of the regulatory bodies and international standards but also provide ease-of-use to patients and users. Packaging systems can include lids (lidstock), pouches, bags, trays and blisters that are used to contain the drugs and medical devices.

General Requirements for Design and Development

Validated Test Methods: Test methods are used to verify the outputs of manufacturing processes. In the case of packaging, some examples of test methods include seal strength.
Robustness of Process: Tests selected for use must adequately address the robustness of the packaging system and process being tested. The rationale for the tests selected for use must be documented in the development protocols.
Design: The design of the blister and lid are properly scoped out, documented and controlled.
Sample Size: Test sample sizes must be based on statistical rationale. The rationale should be documented in the development protocols.

Key Requirements of Medical Packaging

The specific requirements on a given packaging system depend on the classification of medical device. Medical devices are classified based on the application of the devices and the level of risk associated with their use. In general, the level of risk is understood to increase with the (1) duration of use (2) level of invasiveness. Therefore, the packaging requirements for a particular product must be specified correctly and in keeping with the intended use.

High-density polyethylene or HDPE is a popular material that aids in the prevention of microbial contamination. However, the contents and environment must meet microbial standards if a sterile product is being manufactured. The effectiveness of HDPE is based on the amount of very fine filaments and their random orientation makes it an effective barrier.

During the product design phase, the packing configuration must be selected. This selection impacts the equipment and manufacturing technology required in order to deliver the designed barrier system. Most products in a modern manufacturing facility will require a medium to high-volume manufacturing. This is typically driven by market need. If high volumes are not anticipated, a high cycle time may be required to allow the bare minimum number of machines to deliver the throughput required. Storage and shelf life of medical products is also a key concern for the patient and user. In particular, HDPE lidstock can maintain sterility for up to five years. The process of sterilisation involves the controlled release of gases or steam that "penetrates" the packed product but can then quickly escape from the packaging and leave the product sterile and unaffected. Materials must be suitable for the type of sterilisation process.

Inputs

Packaging materials must be compatible with the chosen method of sterilisation, therefore, during the design and development stage, the type of sterilisation must be selected carefully. This is based on regulatory requirements and the capability of the product as well as primary and secondary packaging materials. The requirements with regard to acceptable foreign matter, visual defects, seal strength and integrity criteria must also be developed to form what will be acceptance specifications.

User Requirement Specification (URS) A URS is a requirements document that specifies the intended use of the equipment along with specific operating and process requirements unique to a particular product. The scope of a URS document can be sub-divided into three main sections: (1) installation requirements (2) operational requirements and (3) process requirements.

Installation Requirements: These relate to the type of facility and space available. The footprint and weight of the packaging machine may be a factor for some premises. The customer may also which to procure a packaging solution that is mobile.

Utilities: Typically, electrical and pneumatic supply options are specified in a URS and the machine manufacturer must confirm that the equipment can be successfully operated with the available utilities onsite.

Operational Requirements: Operational requirements may be specific to a particular product or family of products. Some typical examples include:
- Equipment must reach operating parameters from standby within 15 minutes of cold start-up
- It shall be possible to operate the equipment with one person
- Equipment shall be capable of processing a minimum of 20 blisters per minute

Process Requirements: Process requirements can also relate to a specific product or packaging configuration. For example, "the seal shall meet the minimum width specification of 6mm".
While other process requirements are more generic:
- No smudge marks, burn marks or tool marks shall be visible
- Seal areas must be free from creases or any other defects

Outputs

Outputs are essentially the packaging features or attributes that need to be validated and found to be within acceptance levels. For blister packaging, the typical requirements are listed below:

Integrity of sterile barrier
Tensile strength of seal and delamination
Seal width
Cosmetic requirements

Outputs must be considered from the very beginning of a packaging project prior to packaging validation. The choice of materials, equipment and technology can all impact the outcome of the final packaged product. Choosing the wrong materials may cause long delays when issues are discovered or encountered. Choosing the wrong technology, equipment or process may not provide the required capability or necessary quality, especially for regulated products (e.g. medical devices and sterile products).

Sterile Packaging

Packaging materials must be compatible with the chosen method of sterilisation. Sterilisation methods include ethylene oxide, electron-beam, gamma, electron-beam, steam (under controlled conditions) to name but a few. Packaging must provide a high microbial protection and breathability along with acceptable levels of tear resistance and durability.

For sterile medical devices, regulation requirements per EN ISO 13485:2013 include:

"Devices delivered in a sterile state must be designed, manufactured and packed in a non-reusable pack and/or according to appropriate procedures to ensure that they are sterile when placed on the market and remain sterile, under the storage and transport conditions laid down, until the protective packaging is damaged or opened."

"Devices delivered in a sterile state must have been manufactured and sterilised by an appropriate, validated method. Devices intended to be sterilised must be manufactured in appropriately controlled (e. g. environmental) conditions."

"Packaging systems for non-sterile devices must keep the product without deterioration at the level of cleanliness stipulated and, if the devices are to be sterilised prior to use, minimize the risk of microbial contamination; the packaging system must be suitable taking account of the method of sterilisation indicated by the manufacturer."

"The packaging and/or label of the device must distinguish

between identical or similar products sold in both sterile and non-sterile condition".

Stage 2 – Material(s), Equipment and Process technology

Supplier Requirements

Above all, materials must be suitable for the intended use and classification of medical device. Most vendors will operate to a quality management standard such as ISO 9000 or ISO 13485. When dealing with vendors and external suppliers of packaging materials, all medical device manufactures should adopt a vendor approval procedure to specify the supplier requirements.

Materials

Polyvinyl Chloride (PVC)

PVC is a low cost material and suits blister packaging due to its suitability to thermoforming. However, it offers limited barrier protection against moisture and oxygen ingress. PVC blisters provide good protection for physical pharmaceutical solid dose tablets and caplets. PVC sheet thickness is typically between 200µm to 300µm depending on the cavity size and shape. PVC does not provide the highest protection with regards to water vapour ingress. This can be improved by laminating processes using PVDC. To meet suitability for use requirements, PVC formulations need to meet standards such as the US Pharmacopoeia 661, FDA 21 CFR and local regulatory requirements.

PVDC

Polyvinylidene chloride or PVDC is often combined with PVC film by using a lamination technique in order to gain better moisture and oxygen barrier performance. PVDC coated blister films are the most common and prevailing barrier films used for pharmaceutical blister packs.

Cyclic Olefin Copolymers (COC)

Cyclic olefin copolymers (COC) or polymers (COP) can provide moisture barriers to blister packs, typically in multi-layered combinations with polypropylene and polyethylene. Cyclic olefin copolymers have good thermoforming properties even in deep cavities, leading some to use COC in blister packaging as a thermoforming enhancer, particularly in combination with polypropylene or polyethylene.

Lidstock

As previously mentioned, high-density polyethylene or HDPE is a preferred barrier material as it provides excellent protection against water and oxygen ingress. It also can be manufactured to provide good tensile strength offering protection to the product.

An alternative to HDPE lidstock is foil based lidstock. Foil based lidstock can be designed to be heat sealed to polymer blisters such as polypropylene and it suitable for steam sterilisation at high temperatures (over 100°C). Foil based lidstocks also achieve good tensile strength protection for the packaged product.

Equipment and Process Technology

This section describes two approaches to blister packaging of medical devices. The first approach adopted by some manufacturers (especially at initial launch where volumes are relatively low) is for the project or packaging engineer to select a simple manual process. Such a process may consist of the manufacturer receiving pre-formed blisters from a vendor or supplier. The manufacturing only then needs to worry about placing the contents in the blister and sealing it with a lid. The preformed blisters are loaded into each position, the product is placed in the cavity, a lid is placed on the top side of the blister and the sealing process can begin. A more advanced method of blister packaging involves more automated equipment that completes both the forming of the blister and sealing of the lid-to-blister.

Blister sealing is typically completed through pressure heat transfer over a short period of time. Controlled parameters include:
- Seal Temperature
- Seal Time
- Seal Pressure

The seal settings for the above parameters must be determined during process development prior to the commencement of any process validation (OQ and PQ).

Stage 3 - Material Performance and Suitability Testing

The material performance and suitability is demonstrated through testing. This often involves the development of technical reports or the execution of engineering studies to gather the evidence and appropriate rationale to support suitability for use. Prior to any functional or physical testing, test methods need to be validated in advance to ensure they are fit for purpose.

Test Methods

Test methods are used to measure both variable and attribute data that is generated as part of a validation. Variable outputs refer to data that is parametric in nature or continuous. Non-variable data, also known as attribute data is non parametric (such as pass/fail visual inspection)

Variable Outputs

Test method validation must address the following parameters for test methods with variable output:
Accuracy
Precision
Range
Resolution

Attribute Outputs

Test method validation addresses the following parameters for test methods with attribute output:
Effectiveness
Probability of false alarms
Probability of misses

Prior to any test method validation, the test method itself (SOP/procedure) should be available in draft form. The test equipment along with any software should also be qualified and fit for purpose.

Seal Width Measurement

Seal width measurement is a process output that helps to determine the seal integrity post blister sealing. The variable data can be used to monitor the seal quality of blisters and identify any changes in the process that might affect the barrier system.

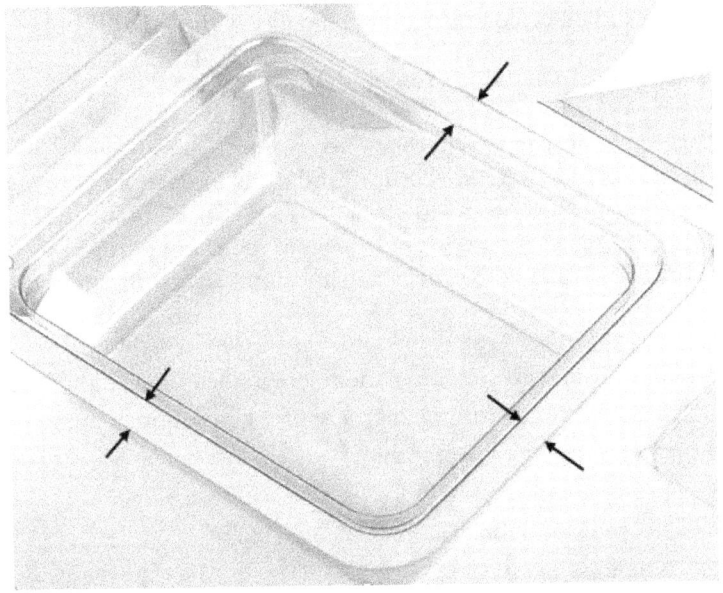

Figure: Seal width

Tensile Testing

Seal strength and seal integrity are critical outputs of the blister sealing process. The worst case sterilisation condition for a material is dependent on the material and the method of sterilisation. However, sealing and subsequent sterilisation at upper and lower worst case conditions should be completed. Tensile testing should be completed in accordance with ASTM F88 or another recognised standard.

Dye Penetration Testing

This test is designed to evaluate the integrity of a sterile barrier system. A blue dye is syringed into a sealed blister with the lidstock intact. The dye should then be allowed come into contact with seal for a defined period of time. Dye penetration testing should be completed in accordance with ASTM F 1929.

Packaging Inspection (Cosmetic)

Packaging inspection should be completed pre and post sterilisation in order to ensure product being sterilised is not damaged or compromised prior to sterilisation. Some typical cosmetic checks are listed below. Packaging inspection requirements should be detailed in an approved specification.

- The entire package must be free of foreign material
- The maximum permitted number of inclusions should be specified along with the max size of the inclusion in mm2
- No smudge marks or burns
- No tool marks
- No voids or bubbles
- No pinholes or tears

Note: For dye penetration, there should be no evidence of penetration across the complete width of the seal.

Bioburden Testing

Bioburden testing will be performed on devices pre-sterilisation to determine the levels of viable organisms that are naturally present on the product or introduced artificially.

Bacterial Endotoxin

Bacterial endotoxin testing is performed in order to test for the presence of bacterial endotoxins of the product. An endotoxin detection test involves testing the liquid sample (or the sample extract) with Limulus Amebocyte Lysate (LAL). LAL is an aqueous extract of the blood cells of horseshoe crabs. LAL forms a clot or changes in colour, depending on the technique used, in the presence of bacterial endotoxin. The test sample is compared to a standard series of Control Standard Endotoxin (CSE) dilutions.

Biocompatibility

Testing is necessary in order to evaluate that the material is biocompatible and appropriate to the intended use of the material/ finished product. Testing ensures the safe application of the device if it is in contact with the body or in used invasively.

Additional Testing

The below testing is normally not a requirement of the packaging validation itself, however, testing may need to be completed during the packaging system development stage or process development in order to ensure the design requirements are met:

Puncture resistance testing is used to measure the toughness of a material punctured via a standard method to determine the relative ability to experience a puncture failure.

Abrasion resistance is a test to determine failure due to rubbing of the product or part of the
package against the primary sterile barrier and the potential to create pinholes or other failures.

Stage 4 - Stability Testing

The purpose of Stability Testing for packaging is to verify that the packaging materials meet requirements over time. Examples of requirements include sterility, functionality, safety, efficacy and visual appearance. Stability testing is also known as "ageing." Stability testing is required for all packaging materials, including blisters, films (lids), cartons and so on. The project team in conjunction with the packaging engineer determines the appropriate testing and time-points and conditions required during testing to verify the packaging system remains fit for purpose over the shelf-life of the product.
In addition to stability testing over real time, stability testing is also conducted in an accelerated manner. This is referred to as

"accelerated" testing or "accelerated ageing".

Testing intervals should be determined based on the shelf life specification of the product in question. The first time point is always t=0 when packaging has just been completed. Sterilised and non-sterilised product should be tested at t=0. Testing must also examine the stability of labels to ensure they remain intact, the material does not crease and the artwork remains legible.

Stage 5 - Packaging Performance Testing

Performance testing the packaging system challenges the acceptability of the entire package system. Performance testing evaluates the interaction between the packaging system and the product in response to the stresses (events) imposed by the production processes and limits, sterilisation processes, storage and transportation environment. The testing is intended to demonstrate that the SBS and protective packaging are adequate to protect the product while maintaining sterility to the point of use. The worst case product configuration is used for this testing.

The following should be considered for inclusion in engineering trials or technical reports:
- Product or representative product is necessary for performance testing.
- Testing should be completed on worst-case product. What is the worst-case product? How was the worst-case product determined?
- What is the worst-case sterilisation process?
- Is the labelling and final packaging reflective of the process/product going forward?

Stage 6- Packaging Validation

Medical Packaging Process Validation

The ultimate aim of process validation for a given packaging system is to demonstrate the manufacturing packaging process is fit for purpose and robust enough to meet the acceptance criteria as set out in product specifications.

Post Equipment Qualification (IQ- Installation Qualification/ OQ- Operational Qualification: Process validation which consists of Process Operational Qualification (OQ) and Performance Qualification (PQ) is required to be completed.

Operational Qualification: Operational Qualification challenges the worst-case process sealing settings to ensure that worst case settings, product seal strengths and the other outputs meet specifications. OQ is typically completed for both high and low worst case conditions e.g. high temperature, high pressure and high seal times versus low temperature, low pressure or low time.

Performance Qualification: Performance Qualification provides a high degree of assurance that the sealing process will consistently produce a packaging system that meets predetermined specifications under normal operating conditions. Any product used in the PQ should be representative of the commercial process going forward.

A minimum of three lots is normally required for the PQ testing for an initial validation. Lots should be based on statistical rational and be reflective of commercial sizes.

Influencing Factors

Process validation aims to prove the consistency of a process under normal operating (anticipated) conditions. Every manufacturing process (however stable) is subject to influencing factors within day-to-day anticipated variation. These influencing factors can be categorised as (1) Worker, (2) Setup, and (3) Material.

For packaging equipment, these factors can influence the performance and consistency of a process and therefore need to be challenged during performance qualification.

A worker or operator can be a source of variation if the process is manual or not fully automated. Different people may have varying levels of expertise, experience and concentration. Even if an operator follows the instructions accurately and complies with standard operating procedures, there will likely be differences in how different operators handle raw materials and the product.

For packaging equipment that requires manual placement of raw materials, multiple operators should be used during the execution of validation builds.

Packaging systems are made up of more than one raw material or component. Whether components are manufactured in-house or supplied externally, they can be subject to variation, even if within the acceptance criteria. Therefore, for packaging validation, a minimum of three distinct lots of each material or component should be used. If multiple tooling is available, set-up can also be a source of variation. In these cases, a minimum number of setups should be completed as part of the validation. If the equipment is intended to run on different days or different shift patterns, the process may be subject to drift. Therefore, the validation should take account of this to ensure normal variation is captured.

Statistical Methods

The packaging process validation OQ and PQ must be

performed using sample sizes and numbers of runs and batch sizes that are based on statistical rationale. A risk based approach should be taken when executing packaging validation.

Sample Size Determination and Sampling Rationale

The number of samples produced during the validation must meet predetermined acceptance criteria that are statistically relevant. This information should be documented in the pre-approved protocol.

Normality

For variable data (continuous data) a test for normality should be completed initially as this determines what type of statistical tool should be used. The normality of variable is verified by completing a normality test using a statistical package such as Minitab© or SPC© If the test returns a P-value $\geq$ 0.01, the data is considered normal. For non-normal data, accepted statistical methods for data transformation or non-parametric analysis should be used.

General Principles of Blister Packaging Validation

- The minimum and maximum critical process parameter set points at which product meeting all critical quality attributes can be manufactured should be defined during process development, ***prior*** to process validation.

- The calibrated range of all critical instruments must be greater than the process range (operating window).

- OQ-P testing will be executed by manufacturing worst case product at minimum process range settings (OQ-P min) and maximum process range settings (OQ-P max) for each critical process parameter. Devices manufactured at worst case minimum OQ-P min and OQ-P max settings must meet acceptance criteria for all critical quality attributes.

- Performance Qualification (PQ) should be manufactured at nominal process settings. Process capability (Cpk) or Process Performance (Ppk) critical quality attributes for each PQ batch.

Variable Print Packaging

This section examines some of the requirements for variable print which is either printed or laser etched onto the surfaces of labels, blisters or cartons.

What is Variable Print?

Variable print is when characters or other shapes or designs printed or laser etched on packaging materials need to change from lot-to-lot or product to product. Examples of variable print include lot/batch numbers, expiry date, date of manufacturing and other unique or variable information required to provide traceability and proper identification of the product.

What Is Fixed Print?

Fixed print is when characters or shapes do not change between lots or batches. The information (characters or shapes) is pre-printed by the component supplier per approved artwork.

Packaging Definitions

Wicking: is the process in which through capillary action, moisture moves from the inside to the surface. During a dye penetration test, wicking can result in a false fail if the dye is exposed to the seal for too long.

Primary Packaging: The labelled inner container in which product is placed and sealed. This generally is the blister pack itself.

Secondary Package: The outer container into which one or more inner containers or "primary packages" are inserted into to form the complete finished product.

Ink Jet Print: applied by a printer that discharges liquid ink, one drop at a time, onto the component.

Laser Etching: "print" is applied by a laser that etches the characters or shapes into the material.

Print and Apply: Labelling method that prints variable print information on a label, then applies the label to a package.

Further Reading

ASTM D1922: Test Method for Propagation Tear Resistance of Plastic Film and Thin Sheeting by Pendulum Method

ASTM D1938: Test Method for Tear-Propagation Resistance (Trouser Tear) of Plastic Film and Thin Sheeting by a Single-Tear Method

ASTM D1242: Resistance of Plastic Materials to Abrasions

ASTM D3420: Pendulum Impact Resistance of Plastic Films

ASTM F1306: Slow Rate Penetration Resistance of Flexible Barrier Films and Laminates

ASTM D1709: Standard Test Method for Impact Resistance of Plastic Film by the Free
Falling Dart Method

Appendix 1

MDR- 2017/745

MDR Chapters, articles and annexes are listed below for reference. Refer to **www.eumdr.com**

CHAPTER I -SCOPE AND DEFINITIONS

Article 1 Subject matter and scope
Article 2 Definitions
Article 3 Amendment of certain definitions
Article 4 Regulatory status of products

CHAPTER II -MAKING AVAILABLE ON THE MARKET AND PUTTING INTO SERVICE OF DEVICES, OBLIG

Article 5 Placing on the market and putting into service
Article 6 Distance sales
Article 7 Claims
Article 8 Use of harmonised standards
Article 9 Common specifications
Article 10 General obligations of manufacturers
Article 11 Authorised representative
Article 12 Change of authorised representative
Article 13 General obligations of importers
Article 14 General obligations of distributors
Article 15 Person responsible for regulatory compliance
Article 16 Cases in which obligations of manufacturers apply to importers, distributors or other persons
Article 17 Single-use devices and their reprocessing
Article 18 Implant card and information to be supplied to the patient with an implanted device
Article 19 EU declaration of conformity
Article 20 CE marking of conformity
Article 21 Devices for special purposes
Article 22 Systems and procedure packs
Article 23 Parts and components
Article 24 Free movement

CHAPTER III - IDENTIFICATION AND TRACEABILITY OF DEVICES, REGISTRATION OF DEVICES AND OF ECONOMIC OPERATORS, SUMMARY OF SAFETY AND CLINICAL PERFORMANCE, EUROPEAN DATABASE ON MEDICAL DEVICES

Article 25 Identification within the supply chain
Article 26 Medical devices nomenclature
Article 27 Unique Device Identification system
Article 28 UDI database
Article 29 Registration of devices
Article 30 Electronic system for registration of economic operators
Article 31 Registration of manufacturers, authorised representatives and importers
Article 32 Summary of safety and clinical performance
Article 33 European database on medical devices
Article 34 Functionality of Eudamed

CHAPTER IV - NOTIFIED BODIES

Article 35 Authorities responsible for notified bodies
Article 36 Requirements relating to notified bodies
Article 37 Subsidiaries and subcontracting
Article 38 Application by conformity assessment bodies for designation
Article 39 Assessment of the application
Article 40 Nomination of experts for joint assessment of applications for notification
Article 41 Language requirements
Article 42 Designation and notification procedure
Article 43 Identification number and list of notified bodies
Article 44 Monitoring and re-assessment of notified bodies
Article 45 Review of notified body assessment of technical documentation and clinical evaluation documentation
Article 46 Changes to designations and notifications
Article 47 Challenge to the competence of notified bodies
Article 48 Peer review and exchange of experience between authorities responsible for notified bodies
Article 49 Coordination of notified bodies

Article 50 List of standard fees

CHAPTER V-CLASSIFICATION AND CONFORMITY

ASSESSMENT SECTION 1 Classification

Article 51 Classification of devices

SECTION 2-Conformity assessment
Article 52 Conformity assessment procedures
Article 53 Involvement of notified bodies in conformity assessment procedures
Article 54 Clinical evaluation consultation procedure for certain class III and class IIb devices
Article 55 Mechanism for scrutiny of conformity assessments of certain class III and class IIb devices
Article 56 Certificates of conformity
Article 57 Electronic system on notified bodies and on certificates of conformity
Article 58 Voluntary change of notified body
Article 59 Derogation from the conformity assessment procedures
Article 60 Certificate of free sale

CHAPTER-VI CLINICAL EVALUATION AND CLINICAL

INVESTIGATIONS
Article 61 Clinical evaluation
Article 62 General requirements regarding clinical investigations conducted to demonstrate conformity of devices
Article 63 Informed consent
Article 64 Clinical investigations on incapacitated subjects
Article 65 Clinical investigations on minors
Article 66 Clinical investigations on pregnant or breastfeeding women
Article 67 Additional national measures
Article 68 Clinical investigations in emergency situations
Article 69 Damage compensation
Article 70 Application for clinical investigations
Article 71 Assessment by Member States
Article 72 Conduct of a clinical investigation
Article 73 Electronic system on clinical investigations

Article 74 Clinical investigations regarding devices bearing the CE marking
Article 75 Substantial modifications to clinical investigations
Article 76 Corrective measures to be taken by Member States and information exchange between Member States
Article 77 Information from the sponsor at the end of a clinical investigation or in the event of a temporary halt or early termination
Article 78 Coordinated assessment procedure for clinical investigations
Article 79 Review of coordinated assessment procedure
Article 80 Recording and reporting of adverse events that occur during clinical investigations
Article 81 Implementing acts
Article 82 Requirements regarding other clinical investigations

CHAPTER VII-POST-MARKET SURVEILLANCE, VIGILANCE AND MARKET SURVEILLANCE SECTION 1 Post-market surveillance

Article 83 Post-market surveillance system of the manufacturer
Article 84 Post-market surveillance plan
Article 85 Post-market surveillance report
Article 86 Periodic safety update report
SECTION 2-Vigilance Article 87 Reporting of serious incidents and field safety corrective actions
Article 88 Trend reporting
Article 89 Analysis of serious incidents and field safety corrective actions
Article 90 Analysis of vigilance data
Article 91 Implementing acts
Article 92 Electronic system on vigilance and on post-market surveillance

SECTION 3-Market Surveillance

Article 93 Market surveillance activities
Article 94 Evaluation of devices suspected of presenting an unacceptable risk or other non-compliance
Article 95 Procedure for dealing with devices presenting an unacceptable risk to health and safety
Article 96 Procedure for evaluating national measures at Union level
Article 97 Other non-compliance

Article 98 Preventive health protection measures
Article 99 Good administrative practice
Article 100 Electronic system on market surveillance

CHAPTER VIII-COOPERATION BETWEEN MEMBER STATES, MEDICAL DEVICE COORDINATION GROUP EXPERT LABORATORIES, EXPERT PANELS AND DEVICE REGISTERS
Article 101 Competent authorities
Article 102 Cooperation
Article 103 Medical Device Coordination Group
Article 104 Support by the Commission
Article 105 Tasks of the MDCG
Article 106 Provision of scientific, technical and clinical opinions and advice
Article 107 Conflict of interests
Article 108 Device registers and databanks

CHAPTER IX-CONFIDENTIALITY, DATA PROTECTION, FUNDING AND PENALTIES

Article 109 Confidentiality
Article 110 Data protection
Article 111 Levying of fees
Article 112 Funding of activities related to designation and monitoring of notified bodies
Article 113 Penalties

CHAPTER X-FINAL PROVISIONS

ANNEXES

ANNEX I GENERAL SAFETY AND PERFORMANCE REQUIREMENTS CHAPTER I GENERAL REQUIREMENTS

CHAPTER II REQUIREMENTS REGARDING DESIGN AND MANUFACTURE

CHAPTER III REQUIREMENTS REGARDING THE INFORMATION SUPPLIED WITH THE DEVICE

ANNEX II TECHNICAL DOCUMENTATION

ANNEX III TECHNICAL DOCUMENTATION ON POST-MARKET SURVEILLANCE

ANNEX IV EU DECLARATION OF CONFORMITY

ANNEX V CE MARKING OF CONFORMITY

ANNEX VI INFORMATION TO BE SUBMITTED UPON THE REGISTRATION OF DEVICES AND ECONOMIC OPERATORS IN ACCORDANCE WITH ARTICLES 29(4) AND 31, CORE DATA ELEMENTS TO BE PROVIDED TO THE UDI DATABASE TOGETHER WITH THE UDI-DI IN ACCORDANCE WITH ARTICLES 28 AND 29, AND THE UDI SYSTEM

ANNEX VII REQUIREMENTS TO BE MET BY NOTIFIED BODIES
ANNEX VIII CLASSIFICATION RULES CHAPTER I DEFINITIONS SPECIFIC TO CLASSIFICATION RULES
CHAPTER I DEFINITIONS SPECIFIC TO CLASSIFICATION RULES
CHAPTER II IMPLEMENTING RULES
CHAPTER III CLASSIFICATION RULES

ANNEX IX CONFORMITY ASSESSMENT BASED ON A QUALITY MANAGEMENT SYSTEM AND ON ASSESSMENT OF TECHNICAL DOCUMENTATION

ANNEX X CONFORMITY ASSESSMENT BASED ON TYPE-EXAMINATION

ANNEX XI CONFORMITY ASSESSMENT BASED ON PRODUCT CONFORMITY VERIFICATION

ANNEX XII CERTIFICATES ISSUED BY A NOTIFIED BODY

ANNEX XIII PROCEDURE FOR CUSTOM-MADE DEVICES

ANNEX XIV CLINICAL EVALUATION AND POST-MARKET CLINICAL FOLLOW-UP

ANNEX XV CLINICAL INVESTIGATIONS
ANNEX XVI LIST OF GROUPS OF PRODUCTS WITHOUT AN INTENDED MEDICAL PURPOSE REFERRED TO IN ARTICLE 1(2)

www.ingramcontent.com/pod-product-compliance
Lightning Source LLC
Chambersburg PA
CBHW070244220526
45465CB00004B/1523